Social and Ethical Issues of Global Pandemics

Africa: Past, Present & Prospects

Series Editors: Toyin Falola, The University of Texas, Austin; and Olajumoke Yacob-Haliso, Brandeis University, Waltham, MA

This series collates and curates studies of Africa in its multivalent local, regional, and global contexts. It aims fundamentally to capture in one series historical, contemporary and multidisciplinary studies which analyze the dynamics of the African predicament from deeply theoretical perspectives while marshalling empirical data to describe, explain, and predict trends in continuities and change in Africa and in African studies.

The books published in this series represents the multiplicity of voices, local and global in relation to African futures. It not only represents diversity, but also provides a platform for convergence of outstanding research that will enliven debates about the future of Africa, while also advancing theory and informing policy making. Preference is given to studies that deliberately link the past with the present and advances knowledge about various African nations by extending the range, breadth, depth, types and sources of data and information existing and emerging about these countries.

Recent and Forthcoming Titles

Social and Ethical Issues of Global Pandemics: A Southern African Perspective edited by Masake Pilisano Harris and Richard Obinna Iroanya

African Perspectives on Global Pandemics and the Challenges of Peace and Security edited by Masake Pilisano Harris and Richard Obinna Iroanya

African Political Economy in the Twenty-First Century: Theories, Perspectives, and Issues edited by Emeka C. Iloh, Ernest T. Aniche, and Stephen N. Azom

Citizenship and the Diaspora in the Digital Age: Farooq Kperogi and the Virtual Community, by Toyin Falola

History, Identity and the Bukusu-Bagisu Relations on the Kenya and Uganda Border, by Peter Wafula Wekesa

Social and Ethical Issues of Global Pandemics

A Southern African Perspective

Edited by
Masake Pilisano Harris and
Richard Obinna Iroanya

LEXINGTON BOOKS
Lanham • Boulder • New York • London

Published by Lexington Books
An imprint of The Rowman & Littlefield Publishing Group, Inc.
4501 Forbes Boulevard, Suite 200, Lanham, Maryland 20706
www.rowman.com

86-90 Paul Street, London EC2A 4NE

British Library Cataloguing in Publication Information Available

Library of Congress Cataloging-in-Publication Data

Names: Harris, Masake Pilisano, editor, author. | Iroanya, Richard O., editor, author.
Title: Social and ethical issues of global pandemics : a southern African perspective / edited by Masake Pilisano Harris and Richard Obinna Iroanya.
Other titles: Africa: past, present & prospects.
Description: Lanham : Lexington Books, 2024. | Series: Africa: past, present & prospects | Includes bibliographical references and index.
Identifiers: LCCN 2023035601 (print) | LCCN 2023035602 (ebook) | ISBN 9781666924831 (cloth) | ISBN 9781666924848 (ebook)
Subjects: LCSH: COVID-19 Pandemic, 2020—Government policy—Africa, Southern. | COVID-19 Pandemic, 2020—Social aspects—Africa, Southern. | COVID-19 Pandemic, 2020—Law and legislation—Africa, Southern. | COVID-19 Pandemic, 2020—Moral and ethical aspects—Africa, Southern.
Classification: LCC RA644.C67 S62283 2022 (print) | LCC RA644.C67 (ebook) | DDC 614.59241440968—dc23/eng/20230731
LC record available at https://lccn.loc.gov/2023035601
LC ebook record available at https://lccn.loc.gov/2023035602

Contents

Preface

COVID-19 pandemic was detrimental with devastating impact on social lives of the citizens, which included negative effects on health, justice, education, democracy, rule of law, business, and employment. The effects thereof persist post-COVID-19, with the possibility to last longer. Governments, in the bid to manage the pandemic and mitigate against its effects, were forced to resort to stringent measures such as lockdown, declaration of a state of emergency, quarantine system, closure of schools, and ban on travel. In addition, governments adopted regulations, some of which were in direct violation of human rights.

This book expounds on these social, legal, and ethical dimensions of COVID-19 in Southern Africa. It analyzes the regulations that were passed during COVID-19 and evaluates the legality of these regulations by measuring them against the Bills of Rights. The book further identifies risks associated with deployment of military in internal territory during pandemics. It is not in question that military agencies were deployed in the fight against COVID-19. These law enforcement agencies were entrusted with the authority to enforce these repugnant regulations and practices. The deployment of the military prompted divided opinions regarding the role of the military. Political scientists, human rights activists, and analysts questioned the military's role as part of the COVID-19 response mechanism. The question of civil-military relations is unsettled. However, it is pertinent to note that military units over the years provided disaster relief in terms of health, education, and other humanitarian efforts when internal service capabilities were insufficient. When armed forces' involvement in domestic affairs occurs, the questions of authorities, military brutality, and firearm use become issues of contention. The consequences included that these measures brought public outcry and were characterized as unlawful, unfair, unethical, unjustified, and discriminatory.

The book further elucidates the incomparability and distinct philosophical approach to security sector governance, law enforcement, and conscious provision of safety and security in a distraught society. This distinction included that people who were in informal settlements, homeless, undocumented, and immigrants, of which the majority were engaged in elementary occupations or casual work purely for survival, were extremely exposed to COVID-19. This was in contrast to the rich, who could afford better medical care and services. For instance, refugees and immigrants were excluded from special funds that were designated to aid the nationals to circumvent the extreme shocks of COVID-19. As a result, those immigrants who relied on craft and elementary occupations and cross-border trading were excluded from earning an income in the host countries, neither were they guaranteed income security in their home countries. As a coping mechanism, some "survival immigrants" relied on goodwill donations or chose "voluntary" deportation.

The book delves deeper into the question of inequality and brings to light the risks associated with informal settings. Informal settlements, reserves, and refugee camps were more prone to the devastating effects of COVID-19 due to conditions such as poor sanitation facilities, living in overcrowded settings, limited access to water supply, minimal job opportunities, limited access to health care, and lack of access to social protection measures. Subsequently, proposed measures to flatten the curve of the pandemic, such as social distancing and washing of hands with running water, were not feasible.

Dr. Masake Pilisano Harris and Dr. Iroanya Obinna Richard

Introduction

Iroanya Obinna Richard
and Masake Pilisano Harris

The outbreak of COVID-19 pandemic was sudden. The spread from its epicenter in Wuhan, China, to other parts of the world was spontaneous and quick, at a breathtaking speed. It pushed the world into unfamiliar territory for the first time in many years. In Africa, as in different parts of the world, societies confronted uncertain times of interruption in quotidian life once taken for granted. Health status of populations across the world plummeted, economies stagnated, and social interactions among people came to a standstill. These disruptions resulted in global economic recession, worsened pre-existing social problems, and interrupted the global food supply chain. Millions of people, particularly on the African continent, faced the risk of starvation.

Governments around the world grappled with how to deal with the existential threat presented by the outbreak of the pandemic to save and preserve lives and humanity from possible extinction on the face of the planet. Fulfilling this natural obligation of states required a full grasp of the epidemiology of the pandemic by both the epistemic community and governments around the world, especially in the midst of conflicting information and disagreements by biomedical experts about the virus. Both scientific knowledge, politics, and buy-in of populations across the world were needed to determine cost and amount of scarce resources necessary to prevent, control, and limit human suffering that the pandemic had unleashed.

An array of quick decisions and countermeasures by governments around the world were projected as essential to preventing, controlling, and managing the outbreak. These measures called for the involvement of all and selfless sacrifice of people across the world for the greater good of humanity. However, the reality of these countermeasures was harsh, as they entailed an upsetting suppression, albeit temporarily, of fundamental human freedoms and social interactions. The decisions and countermeasures against COVID-19 pandemic unfortunately produced losers and winners in different societies across the world. Justifying this outcome, governments and experts argued that, if societies were to survive and return to pre-pandemic normalcy, then swiftly enunciated actions with harsh economic, sociopolitical, and cultural realities were indeed necessary. Urgent calls for faith in governments, patience, and sacrifice were made, and people all the over the world demonstrated their willingness to sacrifice fundamental freedoms in order to save humanity from pandemic threats. However, developments in different countries, especially in Africa, showed there was a limit to which the people were prepared to sacrifice in order to defeat COVID-19. Crippling poverty and realpolitik tested the resolve of the humankind.

Thus, in different countries, for example, Namibia, several COVID-19 control measures were met with much resistance. This book presents a series of discussions on the implications of COVID-19 control measures for democracy, the rule of law, society, and ethics. As the rate of infection, hospitalization, and death increased, societies faced ethical dilemmas and questions around democracy and the rule of law. These conditions brought about by the pandemic provided the motivation for this book. The book represents an attempt to help authorities and society appreciate the extent of the effects of the pandemic and its control measures on people's ways of life. Since this may not be the last of global pandemic outbreak, the questions, reviews, assumptions, and evidence presented in this book are crucial for the present and future generations of humankind and societies.

The book encapsulates and includes contributions that stem from empirical research, and theoretical research. It is organized around two broad themes, namely, the rule of law and ethics, and society and education. The first theme explored the impact of COVID-19 measures on ethics and the rule of law using country case studies. The second theme relates to society and education. The thrusting of ethical dilemmas to the center of discussions of COVID-19 measures in the context of Africa is critical to policymaking. In this regard, Shifotoka Omagano and Masake Pilisano Harris demonstrated how COVID-19 mitigating measures impacted on democracy and the Rule of Law in Namibia. The authors appreciate the efforts of the Namibian government in prioritizing citizens' health over economic interests of individuals, businesses, and the state. Prioritization of health over economics acknowledges the mutuality of people and the state. However, the authors were more concerned about unfairness and discriminatory characteristics of lockdown measures, which restricted freedom of movement within the country and across its national borders. They question the logic of such lockdown measures, which, in addition to restricting freedom of movement, resulted into the cramping of low socioeconomic groups into small spaces in which physical distancing, necessary for preventing the spread of the COVID-19, could not be observed. Equally described as counterproductive were measures that prevented economic activities mostly engaged in by low socioeconomic groups while providing them with insufficient palliatives that could not meet their daily needs. All of these captured the difficulties of respecting ethics in government decision-making processes and balancing health and economic well-being of people during periods of emergency.

Furthering this argument from a criminal justice perspective, Marvin Awarab discusses the facts and myths of ethical leadership within the Namibian justice system during periods of emergency. The author's discussion centers on the process of delivering justice to those who committed lockdown regulation offenses. The thrust of Awarab's discussion is the suspension and gross human rights abuses committed by overzealous agents assigned to effect emergency regulations. He questions the rationale behind delays in the finalization of trials, which worsened during COVID-19 pandemic, singling out absence of ethical leadership within the Namibian criminal justice system as an underlying cause of identifiable flaws. These flaws result in lack of trust in the criminal justice system, as was evident during COVID-19 pandemic.

Accordingly, Malematja Stanley and Eke Udochu looked at legal use of force in the context of COVID-19 enforcement by the police and military from a comparative perspective. With specific reference to Namibia and South Africa, the authors note that ethical questions, rule of law, and legality of actions were evident in police and military activities during COVID-19 pandemic. Whereas law enforcement agents are to enforce the law with due respect to fundamental human rights, there were numerous cases of gross human rights abuses manifested during COVID-19 pandemic in South Africa and Namibia. People who allegedly contravened COVID-19 regulations, like being found outside without cogent reason or requiring permission, were subjected to arrest and inhumane and degrading punishments. The authors posit that observed disproportionate and unreasonable use of force is a threat to right to life, amongst others. As a result, they insist law enforcement should be carried out within the confines of existing laws in times of emergency, such as COVID-19 pandemic. Recorded gross human rights abuses during COVID-19 pandemic gave credence to the contention that law enforcement officers across Africa lack proper understanding of what constitutes reasonable use of force and therefore require regular training on these issues.

Malematja Stanley and Eke Udochu's argument is reinforced by Mabuku Kennedy and Masake Pilisano Harris, who discuss the questions of ethics and internal security in civil-military relations as observed during COVID-19 pandemic in Namibia. The authors specifically focus on military deployment and try to provide answers to questions surrounding the desirability of military deployment in support of civil authorities during periods of emergency. Despite reported shortcomings, they support the deployment of the Namibian Defense Force (NDF) to help the police in enforcing COVID-19 lockdown measures. They reason that defense forces all over the world are trained and equipped to respond to all kinds of emergencies in support of civil authorities and in pursuit of their primary goal of defending the state against military threats. The NDF, they argue, is experienced in doing this, having been deployed in the past to help with rescue operations during floods in different parts of Namibia. Desirability of the NDF deployment, notwithstanding, the authors warn the military risks losing focus on its primary responsibility with frequent deployments to secondary roles in support of civilian authorities.

Furthering this argument from a different angle, Helao Tuhafeni departs from national focus to regional focus in examining security sector governance in times of emergency. The author acknowledges as normal the controversies generated by military deployment in support of efforts to combat COVID-19 pandemic in different SADC countries. In his contribution, governance is broadly used to describe both structures and processes created to ensure adherence to the rule of law, accountability, sense of justice, and security, as well as responsiveness, inclusiveness, empowerment, and participation in the political processes of a country. While the discussion centers on sectoral governance in SADC countries, its applicability to other regional contexts is implicitly stressed.

Helao Tuhafeni's discussion on governance resonates well with Mbetu Gamuchirai and Masake Pilisano Harris who elucidate on sustainable immigration policies and governance discourse. Their discussion focuses on the impact of emergency policies on irregular migration during COVID-19 pandemic in Botswana and South Africa. They stress the unfairness and discrimination inherent in COVID-19 policies and measures in different countries and express concern over their sustainability and impact on Botswana and South African societies. Negative and positive effects of lockdowns, border and business closures, travel restrictions and public transport closures (for non-essential services), and creation of special funds were extensively discussed. Positively, while lockdown measures helped curtail the spread of coronavirus, creation and implementation of "special funds" by South African and Botswana governments, for low-income groups among their populations helped alleviate suffering during the pandemic. On the negative side, however, these measures produced serious adverse effects on survival of the immigrant population, who rely on craft, informal occupations, and cross-border trading for survival.

Lockdown measures prevented survival of the immigrant population from earning incomes in Botswana and South Africa, while exclusion from special fund palliative increased their insecurity and vulnerability in host countries. As a result, the authors call for sustainable immigration governance system nationally and regionally. Governance in the context of the authors' discussion refers to national, regional, and global norms, values, rules, and principles through which immigration issues are managed to ensure respect for human rights, inclusiveness, responsiveness, and participation of immigrant population in meaningful socioeconomic activities of host countries.

Continuing the discussion on the need for sustainable governance in the immigration sector, especially during an emergency period, Ananias Janet, Leonard Emma, and Chikadzi Victor explore the experiences of refugee population during COVID-19 pandemic to draw out critical lessons for social policymaking and social work practice. They posit that drastic measures to curb the spread of the pandemic placed vulnerable groups, such as refugees, at high risk of COVID-19 infection. Refugees, they aver, live in overcrowded settings, have limited access to health care, water supply, and sanitation facilities, they do menial jobs, and have no access to social protection measures. These conditions made it difficult to observe proposed measures to flatten the curve of the pandemic, such as social distancing and washing hands with running water.

The plight of refugees in Namibia, which worsened during COVID-19 pandemic due to several factors, among them unwillingness of states to extend palliative measures beyond their citizens, is blamed on endemic poverty across southern African region. Subsequently, Marvin Awarab looks at deep-rooted poverty and inequalities that exist in societies such as Namibia. The author contends that Namibia is characterized by high levels of poverty and disparity between the rich and the poor. This gap continues to increase over the years, as proven by increase in the number of people living below the poverty line. The outbreak of COVID-19 worsened the situation as economic activities were brought to a halt, albeit temporarily. To improve the economic situation and, by extension, the quality of life for Namibians and refugees, the author proposes revisiting the country's economic policies, especially sustainable development approaches.

Besides negative socioeconomic impacts that widened the gap between the rich and the poor in different African societies, COVID-19 pandemic also severely affected other social dimensions of interactions. In this regard, Shifotoka Monika and Abdallah Ally reinforce the centrality of poverty in their appraisal of the impact of COVID-19 pandemic on Namibian educational system. The temporary closure of schools and institutions of higher learning in order to contain the spread of coronavirus disrupted existing learning system and forced both learners and institutions globally to devise new ways of learning and teaching. Institutions grappled with online teaching and learning platforms in the context of technological inadequacy and lack of access to the Internet for poor learners in the cities and those who reside in rural areas with little or no access to the Internet. The pandemic outbreak revealed the degree of digital divide, lack of resources, and unpreparedness of many African countries, especially Namibia, to transition to new learning modes. Therefore, limited or lack of access to necessary technology infrastructure for both teachers and learners prevented effective delivery of quality educational services and poor academic performance in many cases.

Abdallah Ally and Shifotoka Monika continued the discussion around issues and challenges of digital divide in the drive to provide quality education to Africans from the perspective of Tanzania specifically. They argue that the education industry suffered significantly during COVID-19 pandemic due to sudden change to online modes of teaching and learning. While through online learning institutions in Tanzania were able to support learners to continue their education from a distance, the sudden switch from traditional learning to an e-learning system left behind many students from disadvantaged backgrounds. Digital divide, therefore, presents a significant challenge for those who lack access to information and communication technology facilities and internet connectivity.

From the foregoing, it is evident that this book is a significant contribution to knowledge and understanding of the impact the COVID-19 pandemic had on the rule of law, society, and ethics, as well as socioeconomic development of African states. Discussions and analyses of issues concerning ethics, governance, rule of law, digital divide, irregular migration, and public policy sustainability in times of crisis will resonate with social sciences, political and policy sciences, law, and African studies scholarships.

Chapter 1

The Impact of Mitigating Measures for COVID-19 on the Rule of Law and Democracy in Namibia

Frieda Omagano Shifotoka and
Masake Pilisano Harris

INTRODUCTION

Namibia subscribes to the values of rule of law, democracy, and justice. This is evident in theory and practice; for instance, the Namibian Constitution provides for the principles of democracy, justice for all, and the rule of law. It is important from the onset to note that in Namibia, the Constitution is the supreme law as contemplated in article 1 (6) of the Constitution (Amoo & Skeffers, 2008). The tenets of these values include, but not limited to, a premium on the respect for human rights, upholding rule of law, and promoting democracy. These values and principles were put to test by the incarnation of COVID-19 pandemic. Here, government was summoned to weigh and balance these tenets and values, on one end, and on the other end, limit the same ordained values with the object to curb the spread of COVID-19. On March 17, 2020, a state of emergency was declared by the president. Thereafter emergency regulations were issued. While the measures are justifiable in terms of the Constitution, there was a risk that government may act *ultra vires* and pass unreasonable and unnecessary laws that may allow the abuse or concentration of power. Abuse of power includes negating human rights, rule of law, and democracy. This can have both short-term and long-term impact on the democracy and the rule of law. Some of the measures brought public outcry being characterized as unfair and discriminatory. In addition, there was a risk that states may use emergency powers to combine the executive authority and undermine democracy during the pandemic (Zouey, 2020). This chapter discusses the current and potential impact of the mitigation measures taken by the Namibian government in response to the COVID-19 outbreak on justice, rule of law, and democracy.

THE RULE OF LAW AND DEMOCRACY IN NAMIBIA

Namibia is a democratic state, thus, the presence of the rule of law is reflected in various constitutional provisions relating inter alia to fairness, equality before the law, accountability, separation of powers, respect for human rights, and the supremacy of the Constitution. In addition, the characteristics of a democratic state include but not limited to having a representative elected by the citizens, the protection of human rights, an independent judiciary, and the freedom to join any political party. The presence of the doctrine of the rule of law is a factor that contributes to democracy as it deals with the limits on the powers exercised by government (Ruppel & Ambunda, 2011). Constitutional supremacy is seen in article 1 (6) of the Constitution, and this means that all laws are subject to the Constitution, which is the highest and superior law in Namibia.

Chapter 3 of the Namibian Constitution provides for the Bill of Rights, which contains fundamental human rights and freedoms. According to article 5 of the Constitution, these are to be valued and defended by all the organs of state and persons in Namibia. These human rights in the Constitution are consistent with the provisions of the 1948 Universal Declaration on Human Rights (UDHR). In addition, article 131 of the Constitution prohibits any amendment or repeal that negates the fundamental human rights and freedoms and as such it adds even more value to human rights knowing that the legislature is prevented by the Constitution to pass laws that violate them. According to article 25 (2) of the Constitution, persons whose fundamental rights or freedoms have been infringed have the right to approach the court in order to protect or enforce their rights. Article 10 of the Constitution provides for equality before the law and prevents any discrimination based on "sex, ethnic origin, race, colour, religion, creed or social or economic status." In addition, article 21 provides for the freedom of speech, expression, association, freedom of the media and freedom to peaceful assembly.

The right to a fair trial is one important factor for democracy and the rule of law. In terms of article 12 of the Constitution, this right entails inter alia having access to an independent, impartial, and competent Court, or Tribunal, the trial taking place within reasonable time, accused persons being presumed innocent until proven guilty, being afforded reasonable time and facility to prepare their defense including obtaining a legal representative and judgments in criminal cases being delivered in public unless in the event of minors or because of morality.

The separation of powers is also provided for in article 1 (3) of the Constitution which recognizes the executive, legislature, and judiciary as the three organs of state. The separation of powers is a crucial tool to guarantee and protect the rights of individuals and to prevent dictatorship (Amoo & Skeffers, 2008). This requires the need for checks and balances for the different organs of state to avoid having concentration of power in one organ of state (Ruppel & Ambunda, 2011). The Lower Courts, the High Court, and the Supreme Court, which are under the judiciary in Namibia, are vested with judicial power. The Courts are independent from the executive and legislature in terms of article 78 (2) of the Constitution and are to comply with the Constitution and the law. To further separate the three organs of state, there can be no interference with the judge or judicial officers in the exercise of their duties and functions by Cabinet or Legislative members or any other person.

To further ensure that there is independence of the organs of state, fairness, and accountability, there are checks and balances. Article 18 provides for administrative justice and ensures that there is accountability. This article requires administrative bodies and officials to act in a fair and reasonable manner, and to comply with the requirements imposed by administrative bodies and any relevant laws. Those aggrieved by the action of the aforementioned officials have the right to approach a competent Court or Tribunal for a remedy. This is judicial review of administrative action, which is one of the means to protect individual's rights and prevent the abuse of power (Amoo & Skeffers, 2008). It is important to note that any action taken in terms of any law that eliminates or reduces fundamental rights and freedoms under chapter 3 of the Constitution is invalid in terms of article 25 (1). This relates to any law by a subordinate legislative authority, and action taken by the Executive and Government agencies. A competent Court may order Parliament or the relevant body to correct any defect imposed by such law or set it aside if it is unconstitutional.

There are also bodies and institutions that assist in the protection and enforcement of human rights, ensuring that government is held accountable, the strengthening of the rule of law and democracy. These institutions include the Ombudsman, the Anti-Corruption Commission, the Electoral Commission of Namibia, the Legal Assistance Center, the Judiciary, Namibia Institute for Democracy, the Institute for Public Policy Research, and NamRights. Citizens are aware and have access to these institutions which they approach for assistance and to lodge their complaints. According to the 2018 Ombudsman Annual Report, they received over 3500 complaints, with half of those cases being in respect of maladministration of government institutions and parastatals.

It is even more pleasant to see complaints from rural areas, which shows that even those in rural areas can have access to justice. The presence of democracy and the rule of law is further evident by Namibia's consistent performance in terms of press freedom, being ranked number one in Africa for good press and freedom and 23rd in the world in terms of the 2019 World Press Freedom Index (Reporters without borders, 2019). In terms of the rule of law, Namibia was ranked number one in Africa and number 34 in the world in terms of the World Justice Project 2019 Rule of Law Index. The World Justice Project takes into consideration, *inter alia*, fundamental rights, open government, security and order, and regulatory enforcement as factors in determining the strongest rule of law system (World Justice Project, 2019). Namibia was also amongst the top five countries in Africa with good governance, according to the 2018 Ibrahim Index of African Governance. In terms of political stability performer index Namibia was amongst the top five countries (Africa Country Benchmark Report, 2018). All these rankings and reports reveal the presence of the rule of law and democracy in Namibia and its recognition not only on the African continent, but globally too.

GOVERNMENT COVID-19 MITIGATION MEASURES

The president of Namibia has the authority to declare a state of emergency in terms of article 26 (1) of the Constitution. The state of emergency may be declared in the event of a national disaster, state of national defense, or where there is a public emergency that is threatening the lives of the national or constitutional order. It was on this basis that on March 17, 2020, the president used this authority and declared a state of emergency due to the outbreak of the COVID-19 virus. With the virus spreading all over the world and claiming lives, and Namibia recording positive cases, the threat to the lives of the Namibian people was clear. The effect of a state of emergency, according to article 26 (5) (a) of the Constitution, is that the president shall have the power to make regulations that are necessary for the protection of public safety and the maintenance of law and order. These include the power to suspend the operation of any common law rule or statute or any fundamental right or freedom protected by the Constitution during the period of the state of emergency. The regulations should, however, be consistent with article 24 of the Constitution, which deals with the derogation of fundamental rights and freedoms, which means that conditions that led to the suspension of laws should be reasonably justifiable and have general application.

It was pursuant to article 26 (5) of the Constitution that regulations for the state of emergency were issued. The regulations with measures to be implemented as a means to prevent and suppress the spread of the virus follow some of the guidelines and practices as done in other parts of the world and in terms of advice provided by the World Health Organization (WHO). The regulations were made according to the different stages that the country may migrate to, from stage 1 to stage 4.

Measures Enlisted Under Stage One and Their Impact

The regulations that were applicable in stage 1 of the state of emergency were passed on March 28, 2020. The regulations commenced on March 28, 2020, and ended on April 17, 2020. Although the regulations impacted different aspects of people's lives, the focus is on the provision that directly or indirectly impacts the rule of law, human rights, and democracy. These, among others, included: first, measures related to restrictions on traveling. Traveling from or to restricted areas without a permit was prohibited. For a permit to be granted, the person should be traveling for one of the purposes enlisted in terms of section 6 (5) of the regulations:

(a) purposes of receiving essential medical treatment;
(b) purposes of attending a funeral of a close family member, an acquaintance or a dependent;
(c) purposes of assisting a close family member, acquaintance or dependent who is ill or otherwise suffers from a distressing situation;
(d) any other reason which an authorized officer considers sufficient to warrant the travelling (Proclamation 7 of 2020 Declaration of State of Emergency).

Those traveling for purposes of transporting goods during the course of business, performing essential actions such as enforcement of law or public order, providing health-related services, facilitating the distribution of life necessities, maintenance of necessary infrastructure, and performing other critical services that cannot be reasonably postponed were exempted from obtaining a permit. A person who contravenes these provisions commits an offense and, if convicted, may be liable for a fine not exceeding N$2000 or imprisonment of not more than six months, or both a fine and imprisonment. This provision of the regulations directly limits the freedom to move freely throughout Namibia protected by article 21 (g) of the Constitution.

The entry into Namibia was also prevented for non-Namibian citizens. Drivers transporting goods and officials performing any necessary services relating to the operation of the vehicle or transportation of goods in the course of business were allowed into Namibia. In addition, the regulations empowered the Minister responsible for immigration to issue directives. The prevention of entry into Namibia directly impacts the freedom to leave and return into the country provided for in article 21 (i) of the Constitution.

Second, measures related to judicial proceedings. The regulations were also issued that related to judicial proceedings. The Chief Justice was authorized by section 13 of the regulations to issue directives that suspend, extend, or relax procedures and time periods in the Magistrates or High Court in terms of the Magistrates and the Hight Court Acts and Rules, respectively. It is interesting to note that the directives had force and effect to stay the prescriptions of matters. As a result, directives for the suspension of the operation of certain laws were issued. This was in compliance with article 26 (5)(b) of the Constitution which empowers the President to suspend the operation of any law, statute, or fundamental right or freedom protected by the Constitution for reasonably justifiable purpose during a state of emergency.

The provisions of the directives relating to judicial proceedings during the state of emergency assented on March 31, 2020, related to the following:

(1) *Criminal Matters.* Direction 3 on criminal matters related to accused persons, witnesses, and the cases set down during the lockdown period and was applicable to all criminal matters in all courts. Below are the provisions:

(a) the set down date of all cases set down during the period of the lockdown is to be postponed to a date specified in the Annexure, which Annexure the Chief Justice may amend from time to time, and the applicable order dealing with the status of the accused must correspond to that date;
(b) no accused person, irrespective of his or her status, is required to attend any court proceedings during the period of lockdown: Provided that the following are excluded -
 (i) accused persons brought to court as a first appearance in the Magistrate's Court;
 (ii) accused persons bringing a bail application;
 (iii) accused person who is the appellant in an appeal against the refusal of bail;
(c) no witness subpoenaed or warned to be in any court of law on a date during the lockdown period is required to attend any court proceedings during such period (Directions Relating to Judicial Proceedings During the COVID-19 State of Emergency, Government Notice 90 of 2020).

(2) *Supreme Court, the High Court, and Related Courts.* All superior courts were open to adjudicate urgent and serious matters with limited audience and operational time; for example, courts were between 09h00 and 11h30. (3) *Magistrate's Court*: The Magistrate's Court is open on weekdays between 08h00 and 13h00 for functions of receiving money, receiving and processing documents, and court proceedings in terms of direction 3. In respect of money, it is receiving money for bail payments, traffic fines, maintenance payments and admission of guilt fines. The processing of documents includes those for applications for registration of estates, applications for search warrants, autopsy applications, and protection orders. The court proceedings allowed were in respect of first appearances, urgent bail applications, bail

reductions, and applications for admission into an institution under the Mental Health Act.

(4) *Registry of the Supreme Court, the High Court, and Related Courts.* The Registry of the Supreme Court was only to deal with court process functions and open on weekdays between 09h00 and 11h30. The same working hours were applicable to the Registry of the High Court, Labor Court, Admiral Court, and the Electoral Court. (5) *Suspension of operation of certain laws.* There were provisions of certain laws whose operation was suspended as a result of the state of emergency. This includes the provisions of the Employees' Compensation Act 30 of 1941, Magistrates' Court Act 32 of 1944, High Court Act 16 of 1990, Supreme Court Act 15 of 1990, Arbitration Act 42 of 1965, Prescription Act 68 of 1969, Criminal Procedure Act 51 of 1977, Social Security Act, Labor Act 11 of 2007, Correctional Service Act 9 of 2012, Minerals Prospecting and Mining Act 33 of 1992, Agricultural Commercial Land Reform Act 6 of 1995, and the Electoral Act 5 of 2014. The suspension of the laws came into effect on March 28, 2020, and did not impact actions taken prior to the regulations.

(6) *Exceptions.* Despite the directives, there were proceedings that were not fully or partially impacted by the regulations and directives. This includes the following proceedings in terms of Directive 9, which relate to judicial proceedings during the COVID-19 state of emergency:

(a) applications brought as urgent applications in terms of the rules of the applicable court;
(b) bail applications;
(c) appeals against the refusal of bail;
(d) domestic violence matters;
(e) any case involving children issues;
(f) first court appearance in a criminal case; and
(g) solemnization of marriages in terms of the Marriages Act, 1969. (Act No. 25 of 1969).

Third, measures related to public gatherings. Public gatherings of more than 10 people were prohibited in terms of section 5 (1) of the regulations. This is in respect of people gathered for a common or collective purpose and is not applicable in the event that more than 10 people by coincident find themselves at a specific place. This provision limits the right to liberty provided for in article 7 of the Namibian Constitution and the right to other fundamental freedoms in article 21 of the Constitution such as freedom of association, peaceful assembly, and the freedom to practice religion. A person who organizes or instigates such gathering commits an offense, and upon conviction may be liable for a fine not exceeding N$2000, or imprisonment not exceeding six months, or both a fine and imprisonment. In addition, authorized officers were also given the authority to instruct the dispersant of public gatherings with the use of reasonable measures in terms of section 5 (2) of the regulations.

Fourth, measures related to restrictions on the movement of persons. The regulations also confined people to their place of residence in terms of section 9. The exceptions included if persons were performing critical services, obtaining essential goods or services, getting medical attention, physical exercise, and visiting pharmacies, courts, banks, or food supply stores. The restriction limits the right to liberty in article 7 and the freedoms in article 21 of the Constitution, such as freedom to movement, association, assemble, and move freely in Namibia.

Fifth, measures related to closure of certain businesses. All shops and businesses were to close during the period of lockdown, except for those in the category of critical services. These critical services in terms of annexure B of the regulations include inter alia ambulance, laboratory, dental and other medical services, scientific, disaster management, electricity distribution, portal water, and communication navigation services. In addition, open markets, informal trading businesses, bars, nightclubs, and pubs were also closed because they did not fall within the critical service category. Restaurants, cafes, and coffee shops were allowed to open on a takeaway basis in terms of section 12 (1) (c) of the regulations. This regulation limits the right to practice any profession, occupation, trade, or business in terms of article 21 (1) (j) of the Constitution.

Measures Enlisted Under Stage Two and Constitutive Effects

The regulations for stage two were passed on May 4, 2020, and were to be applicable from that date until June 1, 2020. It is important to note that some of the measures that were in terms of stage one regulations, such as those relating to the prohibition of entry to Namibia, gatherings, and quarantine, remained the same at the time when stage two commenced. In addition, the Chief Justice was still empowered to issue directions in terms of judicial proceedings, and the Ministers were empowered upon the President's authority to issue directives to supplement or amplify the regulations. These directives had similar legal force as the regulations. Thus, the measures that were enlisted under stage two, included but not limited to: first, measures related to schools and higher education institutions. Schools and institutions of higher learning in the country were to remain closed during this stage, but other forms of learning, such as online learning and homeschooling, were allowed as alternatives to face-to-face learning.

Second, measures related to wearing masks. Every person was required to wear a face mask when in a public place, as was contemplated in terms of section 5 of the regulations. Wearing face masks was mandatory. Authorized officers from the police or defense were given the power to instruct a person not wearing a mask to either wear one or leave the public place. Failure to comply with the officer's instruction constitutes an offense, and such person, upon conviction, is liable for a fine not exceeding N$2000, or imprisonment of not more than six months, or both a fine and imprisonment.

Third, measures related to closure of certain businesses. These measures were largely similar to those under stage one regulations. The effect was that businesses that were not categorized as critical services were to remain closed during this period. In addition to the list of prohibited businesses, the operation of cinemas, seminars, conferences, workshops, contact sports and events, casinos and gambling houses, gyms, and entertainment events with more than 10 people was prohibited. Kapana traders were also added on the list of businesses that could operate on a takeaway basis in terms of section 8 (3) of the regulations.

Fourth, measures related to restrictions on the movement of persons. The transportation of goods and persons during the period of lockdown under stage two was allowed within Namibia on condition that measures to prevent the spread of the virus, including the wearing of masks, were observed. This was an obligation that owners and operators of public transportation were required to observe and ensure that preventative measures were put in place and adhered to in terms of section 12 (3) of the regulations.

Measures Enlisted in Terms of Stage Three

The stage two regulations were amended in order to be applicable to stage three from June 1, 2020, to June 28, 2020. And further amendments were made on June 8, 2020, in order for the whole Erongo region to be returned to stage one of the state of emergency regulations. The number of people at public gatherings was increased to 50, and businesses were allowed to resume operation subject to them following the health and hygiene guidelines, including the wearing of masks and observing social distancing as stipulated under section 2 of the regulations. This was also applicable to bars, restaurants, cafes, cinemas, museums, and other traders and businesses that were not allowed to open or where there were restrictions during the first and second stages of the regulations. The easing of the restrictions at least means people were getting back some of their rights and freedoms, such as the right to free movement, association, peaceful assembly, and the freedom to trade and practice their profession.

Measures Enlisted in Stage Four

On June 28, 2020, stage 4 regulations were issued, which were intended to apply to the whole country from June 29 to September 17, 2020. However, because of the high number of cases reported in the Erongo region, the new regulations were not applicable to the Erongo region, which remained under stage 3. During this stage, the measures were more relaxed, with the number of people at public gatherings being increased to 250 in terms of section 6 of the stage four of the state of emergency regulations. However, because of the increase in the number of cases, on the 13th of August 2020 the president announced that the rest of the country went back to stage three, with the Khomas region and Erongo region being on lockdown. This meant that restaurants, bars, and other food traders had to go back to operating on a takeaway basis. In addition, a curfew was introduced between 20h00 and 05h00 where the movement of people was restricted except for those performing critical services. This shows how unpredictable things can be during a pandemic. At the end of the state of emergency on September 17, 2020, the Public and Environmental Health Act 1 of 2015 became applicable to regulate COVID-19 measures going forward to inter alia promote health, prevent diseases, provide early detection of diseases protect the public from public health risks.

ANALYSIS OF THE IMPACT OF THE MITIGATION MEASURES ON JUSTICE

As part of the research, a survey was shared on the mitigation measures in Namibia. A total of 13 responses were received from officials working for the Judiciary, Ministry of Justice, Law Reform and Development Commission, and other officials who chose not to disclose their work. The aim was to determine the type of measures put in place in the workplace and the impact of such measures, if any, on rule of law and governance. Officials who participated in the survey included legal officers, legal practitioners' interpreters, and others who did not disclose their positions. Below are some of the questions and responses from the participants.

Most of the responses to the question, "What challenges did you encounter in your work due to COVID-19?" identified online working and postponement of cases as some of the challenges that were experienced. In respect to online working, it was apparent that online working was difficult to implement as not everything could be done online. For instance, not all courts in Namibia are equipped with and have access to Electronic Justice System (EJS); hence, it was not possible for litigants and lawyers to file documents online and they needed to attend to filling at the courts. It was also difficult to serve documents such as summons and correspondences to accused persons and defendants because of the measures in place. Whereas, in relation to the challenges associated with the postponement of cases, the responses revealed that trials could not proceed and cases had to be postponed. This meant that witnesses, accused persons, plaintiffs, defendants, and legal practitioners could not attend to court matters.

Another question is to determine the impact of COVID-19 on plaintiffs, defendants, and accused persons. The responses identified several rights that were impacted, among others: trial within reasonable, inmate visit, and right to justice. On the issue of the Right to trial within a reasonable time: one of the challenges of the pandemic identified by participants on litigants is their right to fair trial as provided for in article 12 of the Constitution. This was because trial dates had to be postponed, which caused a delay in the finalization of cases, which directly impacted the right to trial within a reasonable time. The postponement of cases also meant that witnesses could not testify, and legal practitioners and prosecutors could not consult and prepare witnesses for trial. This also impacted accused persons' rights to liberty for those who were in custody or holding cells. For the provision made, that is, for accused persons who needed to apply for bail on the basis of urgency, this was done in terms of written submissions only. This means that accused persons and or their legal practitioners did not get the opportunity to cross-examine witnesses, which then can impact the outcome of the case. In addition, this puts financial burdens on both parties involved because of further postponement of cases, especially for those with legal representatives.

On the issue of visitation of inmates, it is important to note that the directives under the regulations that suspended the operation of certain laws also impacted the visitation rights of inmates and prisoners, who, apart from already being deprived of their liberty, could not see their family members and friends and could also not receive food from them.

The other challenge that was noted in the responses was a claim that discouraged plaintiffs from opening cases. The participants revealed that there was a decline in new cases, with one of the contributing factors being that plaintiffs and complainants were discouraged from opening cases considering that during the pandemic trials were being postponed. This also meant that it was difficult for police officers or court officials to serve summons or arrest accused persons because of the restrictions in terms of the regulations. In addition, there was an increase in withdrawal of cases to avoid going to public places, which were considered breeding grounds for COVID-19.

The other question was to solicit participants' views on the impact of COVID-19 on the justice system. Several responses identified the backlog of cases as the biggest challenge that the justice system was faced with. The indication was that because of the disruption in work and the postponement of cases, there was a significant delay in the finalization of cases. This caused cases to pile up and even bigger backlog of cases in courts. The delay impacted the operation of the court, and in the long run, it impacts the whole justice system. Further that the non or partial operation of the courts placed enormous pressure on the litigants. This means the justice system was negatively impacted by the state of emergency regulations, which then directly and indirectly impacted the judiciary as an organ of state as provided in article 1 (3) of the Constitution.

In summary, the responses presented above strongly demonstrate that the right to a fair trial for accused persons and parties in both civil and criminal proceedings, as stated in article 12 of the Constitution was impacted by measures imposed as a result of the state of emergency. One such right in terms of article 12 (1) (b) is the right to trial within a reasonable time. Because of the postponement of trials and for courts only dealing with special matters such as urgent bail applications, which took place by means of affidavits, the right to have a speedy trial was deprived, and for those in custody, their right to liberty was also further deprived. Even in such exceptions, evidence was limited because witnesses were not testifying, and oral evidence is one of the most important types of evidence that has been used in our courts. The important characteristic of the principle of orality in terms of evidence is that it requires evidence to be presented orally, in the presence of the public and the parties to the dispute, and subject to cross-examination (Broodryk, 2020). This was, however, not entirely possible because of the directives under the regulations due to the state of emergency.

The right to a fair trial also comprises a public hearing and judgment being delivered in public in terms of article 12 (1) (a) of the Constitution and because of the regulations, this was not done. This also impacted the principle of democracy in that it was difficult for the media to report on cases and for the public to scrutinize the judgments. It is notable that the regulations prohibited or imposed travel restrictions. The travel restriction impacted the access to justice, i.e., trials not starting, postponement of cases, and no contact with different parties involved in civil and criminal cases, such as witnesses, investigators, prosecutors, and legal practitioners, all of which affects access to justice. This burden was even worse for courts that do not have the capacity to use the EJS online system, which means that there was no progress in the cases.

COLOSSAL IMPACTS OF COVID-19 ON THE RULE OF LAW AND DEMOCRACY

There are several characteristics of a democratic state, among others. First, the citizens have the right to vote, the freedom to form or join any political party of their choice, and to influence the structure and policies of government. These democratic rights are provided for in terms of article 17 of the Constitution. Unfortunately, these rights were limited by the regulations on

COVID-19, namely, the suspension of the operation of Part 1 and 2 of Chapter 5 of the Electoral Act 2014, which deals with preliminary arrangements for the conduct of elections. With the regional and local authority elections that were scheduled to take place in November 2020, the ECN had to ensure that it was prepared, and the elections were required to take place in compliance with COVID-19 measures.

The boundary clarification exercise, which identifies and verifies registration points and ensures that voters registered under wrong constituencies were issued with correct voters' cards initially scheduled to take place in March 2020, had to be postponed, and the supplementary voter's registration could only take place from September 7 to 15, 2020, because of the pandemic (ECN, 2020). This and other developments in terms of the pandemic also impacted the activities such as public consultations, supplementary voters' registration, and nominations of candidates, which preceded the November 2020. Despite the interruption of the election process by the pandemic and delay of some activities, the elections were scheduled for November 25, 2020, to avoid additional costs, legal implications, and amendments to laws as consequences of a postponement (Iikela, 2020).

Secondly, an issue that is noteworthy when dealing with democracy and rule of law is fundamental freedoms. There are many rights and freedoms that were limited and impacted directly or indirectly in different ways as a result of government response measures to the COVID-19 pandemic. These included, inter alia, (a) the right to a fair trial because of the postponement of trials or the limitation of the number of people required to be present in court. (b) the right to education under article 20, which requires the state to provide reasonable facilities for this right to be effective for every resident within Namibia. The right to education could not be achieved because not all learners had access to online learning or had guardians who could assist with homeschooling. (c) The right to freedom of the media was also impacted because of the reduction in the number of journalists and other media practitioners who were able to cover government briefings and the inability and limitation in terms of having access to courts to report on court cases, especially during stages one and two of the regulations. This includes the works of investigative journalism that required travelling and interviews. (d) The restrictions on the number of people in public gatherings also directly impacted the freedom to practice religion and the freedom to peaceful assembly, including demonstrations and associations. (e) The travel restrictions directly limited the right to freely move in Namibia and the right to leave and return to Namibia. (f) The measures also had a socioeconomic impact as it limited the right to practice any profession or carry out any business or trade except for those who provide essential services; the impact was greater during stages one and two of the regulations. This led to a loss of income and loss of employment for many Namibians.

Thirdly, is the question of international diplomacy. The measures do not only impact democracy and the rule of law in Namibia; however, they directly and indirectly impact different areas beyond the borders. An example is the restriction on travel and the limitation of public gatherings impacted international diplomacy and the ability for representatives to attend, discuss, and negotiate on issues of regional and international concerns. Although there may be alternatives, such as online platforms, to having meetings, this was a challenge taking into consideration the different time zones, and it took away the opportunity to talk to and discuss with partners and rivals before making decisions. In addition, restrictions on the entry into Namibia by non-residents and those who are not citizens also had negative impact on migration and worse refugees and asylum seekers.

Fourth is the issue of human rights limitations. There are limitations to the human rights and freedoms in terms of article 22 of the Constitution. However, any law providing such limitations should comply with the following requirements:

(a) be of general application, shall not negate the essential content thereof, and shall not be aimed at a particular individual;
(b) specify the ascertainable extent of such limitation and identify the article or articles hereof on which authority to enact such limitation is claimed to rest.

The state of emergency is a form of limitation to human rights and freedoms; as such, it has a direct impact on democracy and rule of law. For it to be a limitation under article 22 of the Constitution, the above-mentioned requirements should be met. In looking at the provisions of article 26 of the Constitution, which provides for the declaration of a state of emergency, it can be concluded that it was done in compliance with article 22. This is because, as provided for in article 22 (a) of the Constitution, the state of emergency, the laws and regulations that consequently followed were not targeted at individuals or groups of people, and the aim of the state of emergency and the regulations was to stop and prevent the further spread of a global pandemic. In terms of article 22 (b) of the Constitution the extent of the limitation must be specified and the article in terms of which the authority to impose such limitation is derived from. The declaration of the state of emergency due to COVID-19 pandemic specifically stipulates that it was done in accordance with article 26 (1) of the Constitution. In addition, the regulations stipulate the date of commencement, the application, and the duration, which is sufficient to ascertain the extent of the application of the regulations. Hence, it can be concluded that the state of emergency and, consequently, the regulations comply with the requirements of article 22 of the Constitution.

The violations of human rights during the pandemic were a threat to democracy. For example, during stage one of the lockdown, the military, police, and municipal police were dispatched around the country to ensure compliance with the regulations and maintain order. However, there were complaints of disproportionate use of force and violation of human rights by these authorized officers who assaulted civilians and damaged their goods and properties, with videos of the cruel acts shared on various social media platforms (Mbathera, 2020). This is not only abuse of authority, however, but also a violation of the individual's human dignity and amounts to inhumane and degrading treatment. Considering that the courts were not fully operational because of the regulations, this made it even worse in terms of having access to justice for the protection and enforcement of fundamental human rights. Hence, it is not the limitation on fundamental human rights and freedoms that constitutes human rights violations; however, it is the acts of those responsible for the compliance of the regulations, such as the police and military, that constitute human rights violations.

POST-COVID-19 IMPLICATIONS

The struggle for democracy continues after the pandemic. As the world got back to what was branded as the new normal, the government in Namibia also followed suit by relaxing the imposed measures. However, the impact of the COVID-19 pandemic on democracy continues even post the pandemic. One of the challenges is the backlog of cases that the judiciary deals with because of the pandemic, which is reflected in the reduction in the number of cases that the Courts were able to finalize during the period of the state of emergency. The average of finalized criminal cases in the High Court's Main Division during the 2020 legal year was 30 percent and 25 percent for the Northern Local Division and the Lower courts could only finalize 20 percent of the cases on the rolls (Dgru, 2022). This has added to the already-existing backlog of cases that the Judiciary had before the pandemic. Post-COVID-19, the courts must deal with both new cases and the old ones that could not proceed during the pandemic.

On a lighter note, the measures imposed by the COVID-19 pandemic also forced litigants and lawyers to make use of the E-Justice platform to file documents in respect of civil proceedings and electronic case management system. The platform benefits legal practitioners, the courts, judges, and litigants as they can directly make entry of documents required during the litigation process, status reports, and court orders (Judiciary, 2018). The E-Justice platform helps improve efficiency in the court process, therefore enhancing access to justice. There is an opportunity for the Judiciary to extend the system to criminal cases, as it is currently applicable to civil matters; this can reduce paper-filling procedures and help improve efficiency in the criminal justice system. Further, Parliament passed the Access to Information Act 8 of 2022 on December 28, 2022, which will have an impact on the right of access to information held by public and private entities and will therefore help improve democracy in the Country as it impacts the right to freedom of speech and expression and freedom of the media in article 21 of the Constitution and can also help improve administrative justice under article 18. In the preamble of the Act, the objectives of the Act are inter alia to appoint an independent and impartial information commissioner, to provide for the right to access information, and to facilitate the promotion, keeping, and organization of information in a transparent, accountable, and good governance manner (Access to Information Act 8 of 2022).

The presence of the rule of law and democracy in Namibia continues to improve and is still recognized as one of the top countries in Africa in terms of democracy. In terms of the 2020 Mo Ibrahim Index on Governance, Namibia is ranked 7th in the world for overall governance. Further, in respect of the World Justice Project, Namibia is ranked 46th in the world and 3rd in the region (World Justice Project, 2022). Further, the presence of democracy and the rule of law is evident by Namibia's consistent performance in terms of press freedom, being ranked number one in Africa for good press and freedom and 18th in the world in terms of the 2022 World Press Freedom Index (Reporters Without Borders, 2022), which is a higher ranking compared to the 2019-2020 report. In respect of the categories rated include fundamental rights, absence of corruption, civil justice, regulatory enforcement, order and security, and criminal justice. Other institutions, such as the Ombudsman, continue to serve the public and assist citizens to protect their human rights, and promote fair and effective administration. Despite the COVID-19 challenges, the office of the Ombudsman continues to perform and ensure that administrative bodies and officials are held liable, and during 2021/2022, 84 percent of the 2880 cases reported to the Ombudsman were resolved, compared to 88 percent during the 2018/2019 annual year (Ombudsman 2021/2022 Annual Report). Most of the reported complaints related to maladministration, which include human rights violation, administration of justice, police conduct and failure to act, compensation, and government ministry conducts (Ombudsman 2021/2022 Annual Report). The institutions with the highest complaints during the period were the police, the judiciary, the correctional services, and the Ministry of Health and Social Services.

RECOMMENDATIONS

The impact of the measures of the state of emergency on the rule of law and democracy is evident, with courts unable to fully operate during the pandemic and accused persons rights to a fair trial, amongst others, being negatively impacted due to the postponement of cases, the lack of witnesses to travel to testify in court because of travel restrictions. The limitations on the freedom of association, taking part in political activities, freedom of the press, freedom of peaceful assembly that characterize a democratic state also have both short-term and long-term effects on democracy. Hence, the government needs to review the current measures and policies relating to emergencies and come up with a framework that can be used to deal with future pandemics and global crisis. One of the things exposed during pandemic was the lack of the necessary infrastructure in terms of technology, including equipped courtrooms and virtual systems that allow aggrieved persons to have access to justice without direct contact where possible. The Supreme Court had its first virtual court hearing for a labor appeal matter during the pandemic, and this can be a new way of enhancing access to justice and ensuring that the court process is expedited (Jantjies, 2020).

In addition, the government should take advantage of the pandemic as an opportunity to review its policies and make changes to the legal system. Government can also make use of the United Nations (UN) guidelines such as the UN Rule of law, support, and Guidance Notes on ensuring access to justice in the context of COVID-19. The guidelines provide policymakers with important notes in terms of preparation, response, and recovery in ensuring access to justice in the context of COVID-19 pandemic. Furthermore, the government should also have a review of its performance during the state of emergency so that it can be better prepared for future emergencies.

CONCLUSION

One cannot deny that COVID-19 pandemic claimed the lives of many, weakened the public health systems of governments, and burdened the economy. It also impacted democracy in many states, and Namibia is no exception. The measures taken by each sovereign state were supposed to take into consideration both the short-term and long-term effects and put into consideration the recovery and what is called the new normal post-COVID-19 pandemic. Measures taken by the Namibian government limited fundamental human rights, including the rights to fair trial, freedom of association, freedom of assembly, freedom of movement, and freedom of the press, which were some of the fundamental rights and freedoms directly impacted by the measures.

Government should ensure that the measures imposed as a result of the state of emergency are necessary, reasonable, and legal so that there will not be an abuse of power and in order for democracy and the rule of law not to be weakened.

REFERENCES

Access to Information Act 8 of 2022-Namibia.

Agricultural Commercial Land Reform Act 6 of 1995 – Namibia.

Amoo, S. & Skeffers, I. The Rule of Law in Namibia. (2008). Retrieved from https://www.kas.de/c/document_library/get_file?uuid=bec5a239-1da4-5257-c471-cf1a73e35142&groupId=252038

Arbitration Act 42 of 1965 – Namibia.

Broodryk, T. The Erosion of the Principle of Orality in South African Civil Procedure: Fact or Fiction? (2014). Retrieved from http://specjuris.ufh.ac.za/sites/default/files/Broodryk.pdf

Correctional Service Act 9 of 2012 – Namibia.

Criminal Procedure Act 51 of 1977 – Namibia.

DGRU. Impact of COVID-19 on the Administration of Justice in Namibia, Malawi and South Africa. (2022). Retrieved from https://www.judgesmatter.co.za/wp-content/uploads/2022/05/COVID19-Report_-State-of-Judiciary-in-Malawi-Namibia-and-South-Africa-2022.pdf

Directions Relating to Judicial Proceedings During the COVID-19 State of Emergency, Government Notice 90 of 2020, Published in Government Gazette no. 7160 on 31 March 2020 Assented to on 31 March 2020 Commenced on 31 March 2020.

Electoral Act 5 of 2014 – Namibia.

Electoral Commission of Namibia. Supplementary Registration of Voters 07th – 15th September 2020. (2020). Retrieved from https://www.ecn.na/supplementary-registration-of-voters/

Employees' Compensation Act 30 of 1941 – Namibia.

High Court Act 16 of 1990 – Namibia.

Iileka, S. November Polls to Go Ahead Amid Covid-19. *The Namibian Newspaper.* (22 June 2020). Retrieved from https://www.namibian.com.na/201933/archive-read/November-polls-to-go-ahead-amid-Covid-19

Jantjies, N. Virtual Court Hearings: A New Era in the Namibian Judicial System. *The Namibian Newspaper*. (2020, August 7). Retrieved from https://www.namibian.com.na/93499/read/Virtual-Court-Hearings-A-New-Era-in-the-Namibian-Judicial-System

Labour Act 11 of 2007 – Namibia.

Magistrates' Court Act 32 of 1944 – Namibia.

Mbathera, E. Two Young Men Reported a Case of Assault with Intent to Cause Body Harm against Members of the Namib Desert/Operation Covid-19 Last Tuesday. *The Namibian Newspaper*. (2020, May 18). Retrieved from https://www.namibian.com.na/200996/archive-read/Two-men-claim-police-brutality

Minerals Prospecting and Mining Act 33 of 1992.
Mo Ibrahim. Mo Ibrahim Index 2018. (2020). Retrieved from https://iiag.online/data.html?loc=NA&meas=GOVERNANCE&view=graph&subview=score&range-1from=2010&range1to=2019
Ombudsman. Ombudsman Namibia Annual Report 2018. (2019). Retrieved from https://www.ombudsman.org.na/wp-content/uploads/2019/09/2018-report.pdf -
Ombudsman. Ombudsman Namibia Annual Report 2021/2022. (2022). Retrieved from https://ombudsman.org.na/wp-content/uploads/2022/11/Annual-Report-2021_22_compressed.pdf
Prescription Act 68 of 1969 – Namibia.
Proclamation 7 of 2020 Declaration of State of Emergency: National Disaster (Covid 19) – Namibia.
Public and Environmental Health Act 1 of 2015-Namibia.
RSF. 2020 World Press Freedom Index. (2020). Retrieved from https://rsf.org/en/ranking
RSF. 2020 World Press Freedom Index. (2021). Retrieved from https://rsf.org/en/index
Ruppel, O. & Ambunda, L. *The Justice Sector and The Rule of Law in Namibia: Framework, Selected Legal Aspects and Cases*. (2011). Retrieved from https://www.nid.org.na/images/pdf/democracy/Framework_Namibian_Justice_Sector.pdf
Social Security Act – Namibia.
Supreme Court Act 15 of 1990 – Namibia.
United Nations Office on Drugs and Crime. *Access to Justice & COVID-19*. (2020). Retrieved from https://www.un.org/ruleoflaw/wp-content/uploads/2020/06/Ensuring-Access-to-Justice-in-the-Context-of-COVID-19.pdf
World Health Organization. WHO Director-General's Opening Remarks at the Media Briefing on COVID-19 11 March 2020. (2020). Retrieved from WHO Director-General's opening remarks at the media briefing on COVID-19 – 11 March 2020.
World Justice Project. World Justice Project Rule of Law Index 2019. (2019). Retrieved from https://worldjusticeproject.org/sites/default/files/documents/WJP_RuleofLawIndex_2019_Website_reduced.pdf
World Justice Project. World Justice Rule of Law Index 2022. (2022). Retrieved from https://worldjusticeproject.org/rule-of-law-index/global/2022/Civil%20Justice/
Zouey, A. Covid-19 and The Rule of Law. *The Global Observatory*. (2020). Retrieved From https://reliefweb.int/report/world/covid-19-and-rule-law

Chapter 2

Ethical Leadership in the Namibian Criminal Justice System

Is It a Fact or Myth?

Awarab Marvin

INTRODUCTION

The practice of ethics is fundamental to the field of criminal justice. Ethics must be upheld at all levels of law enforcement to guarantee that people are treated fairly and in compliance with their legal rights. There have been numerous allegations on social media and various other platforms that some of the members of the criminal justice system act in an unethical manner and do not provide services efficiently. Whether these allegations are founded or not is a matter of debate. This chapter thus provides a discussion on what ethics is and how it functions in the criminal justice system from the Namibian perspective.

Today's world is undergoing a massive ethical shift that must embrace all humans. Ethics, also known as moral philosophy, is a branch of philosophy that is used to study complete human behavior and ways of being. It is a systematic approach to understanding, analyzing, and differentiating between right and wrong, good and bad, commendable and deplorable, as it relates to the welfare of conscious beings (Holmes, 1998). On the other hand, legal ethics is defined as the appropriate standards that are required of a person within the legal profession when exercising their duties.

Amongst other things, ethics provides us with a way to make moral choices when we are uncertain about what to do in a situation involving moral issues. In the process of everyday life, moral rules are desirable, not because they express absolute truth but because they are generally reliable guides for normal circumstances (Singer, 1995).

TYPES OF ETHICAL ENQUIRY

Within the study of ethics, there are three branches, namely: Normative ethics, meta-ethics, and lastly, descriptive/applied ethics. The first approach attempts to inquire how humans should behave, what ought to be done in certain circumstances, and further investigates the type of character one should have. Common morality forms part of this approach, and it consists of normative beliefs and behaviors that the members of the community generally agree about. For example, while robbing a bank and murder are classified as common morality, the same cannot be said about abortion because people have conflicting opinions and beliefs about its rightness and wrongfulness (Singer, 1995).

Second, we have meta-ethics. This approach does not concern itself with what ought to be done but focuses on understanding the language of morality through an analysis of ethically related concepts and theories, such as the meaning of what is said or done. For example, determining the meaning of a good nurse-patient relationship would be the meta-ethical analysis of a nurse.

Descriptive ethics, which is the last approach, is a scientific approach rather than a philosophical ethical enquiry. This approach is used when researchers want to describe what people think about morality. Research that analyzes how nurses behave when telling their patients the truth about chronic diseases is a practical example of this approach (Singer, 1995).

ETHICS AND THE CRIMINAL JUSTICE SYSTEM

The criminal justice system comprises various agencies whose role is to uphold the law for the welfare of all citizens. Its aim, therefore, is to deliver justice by convicting the guilty party while protecting the innocent party. The criminal justice system thus has a duty to detect crime, carry out court orders, and supervise custodial punishment (Shakil, 2015, pp. 332–342). A question that one can pose is whether ethics and ethical conduct have a place in the criminal justice system. Ethics are fundamental in detecting crime, bringing it to justice, and carrying out the orders of court, such as collecting fines, and supervising community and custodial punishment (Shakil, 2015, pp. 332–342).

Ethics and the rule of law are key aspects of democracy, and thus, in upholding the constitutional order of democracy, freedom, and justice, it is imperative that people of all spheres of life conduct themselves ethically. More importantly, those involved in a criminal justice system are entrusted to uphold justice and the role of law and should therefore act ethically. In Namibia, like most other jurisdictions, various stakeholders play a role in ensuring that justice prevails. Relevant stakeholders operate collectively in the sense that the duties of one office, that is, the office of the prosecutor, depend on those of the other, that is, the office of the investigator in the police department, to undertake a comprehensive investigation. Although a prosecutor is not limited to singlehandedly gather evidence and taking the necessary steps that will assist him or her to pursue the case through trial, conducting proper investigations by the investigator makes the process less complex. Magistrates or judges become pivotal persons at the last stage of the criminal justice system as they determine the innocence or guilt of the accused person based on the evidence presented in court with viva voce or by means of a written testimony.

The importance of ethics in the criminal justice system is found in the fact that ethics provides a set of rules and guidelines for criminal justice practitioners. The rules of ethical judicial conduct in Namibia set out ethical rules such as independence, impartiality, integrity, propriety, and equality. Some of the rules are discussed in this chapter as it applies to ethical leadership. No functionary of the criminal justice system is exempted from complying with ethics.

FUNCTIONARIES IN THE CRIMINAL JUSTICE SYSTEM

As mentioned in the introductory paragraphs of this chapter, there are various functionaries: the police officer, the prosecutor, the presiding officer, and the prison warden involved in the criminal justice system.

The Namibian Police Force

Ethics can influence police behavior in various ways, starting with how the police interact with the community and how the community interacts with the police. When a police officer acts ethically, the ripple effect is that the community is more likely to be ethical when dealing with them, and this will result in them working together to prevent crimes. In the case of *Ushinge v Government of the Republic of Namibia* [2020] NAHCMD 341 the plaintiff was unlawfully and wrongfully taken into custody by police officers. Thereafter, he was detained at Katutura Police cells for 55 hours without any proper detention documents and without appearing before a court of law. The conduct of the police officers was clearly unethical because the letter of the law states in Article 11(3) of the Constitution as follows:

> All persons who are arrested and detained in custody shall be brought before the nearest magistrate or other judicial officer within a period of forty-eight (48) hours of their arrest or, if *this is not reasonably possible, as soon as possible*

> *thereafter*, and no such persons shall be detained in custody beyond such period without the authority of a magistrate or other judicial officer [my emphasis].

Police officers are empowered by the government to enforce law and to ensure public order through the legitimized use of force (Newham, 2015, pp. 39–48). Furthermore, police officers are allowed to intervene in the lives of citizens, however, under limited and carefully controlled circumstances subject to the rule of law (Newham, 2015, pp. 39–48). Additional duties of police officers include to intervene when a crime has been committed or there is imminent threat or likelihood that a crime is about to be committed. The Namibian police force is a creature of statute and was established in terms of the Police Act 19 of 1990. The preamble of the Police Act in particular sets out the purpose of the Act. It states that:

> The Act is meant to provide for the establishment, organization and administration of the Namibian Police Force; to regulate the powers and duties of the Force and to prescribe the procedures in order to secure the internal security of Namibia and to maintain law and order; to regulate the discipline, appointment, promotion and discharge of members of the Force; and to provide for incidental matters.

Its primary functions include the investigation of any offence or alleged offence, the prevention of crime, and the protection of life and property. (Section 13 (a)(c) of the Police Act 19 of 1990.) Section 14 of the Act sets out the powers and duties of the members of the police force and states that:

> Every member shall be competent to serve or execute any summons, warrant or other process authorized by law, and if the member who originally has had to serve or execute the summons, warrant or other process, is unable to serve or execute such summons, warrant or other process, such summons, warrant or process may be served or executed by any other member, and every such last-mentioned member shall have the same rights, powers and authorities for and in the service or execution of such summons, warrant or process which the member had who originally has had to serve or execute the summons, warrant or other processes.

The police are charged with the power to arrest persons accused of committing an offense, and the law prescribes the way an arrest may be affected. In terms of section 39(1) of the Criminal Procedure Act, 15 of 1977, arrest may be affected by actually touching the body of the person sought to be arrested. A police officer is empowered to use reasonable force to effect arrest if the circumstances so require. This may normally happen in instances where the person to be arrested resists the arrest. The use of force is permitted in terms of the law; however, police officers are not permitted to mistreat accused persons.

Although the right to liberty of the accused person is deprived as a consequence of such an arrest, the fundamental human rights and freedoms of such a person are not taken away. Article 7 of the Namibian Constitution supports these claims, as it states that "no person may be deprived of personal liberty except according to procedures established by law." This means that the arrest and subsequent detention of an accused person must be done according to the procedures. A police officer who acts outside the scope of his or her mandate or who unnecessarily inflicts harm on the person sought to be arrested may invite criminal charges or delictual claims against him or herself. Furthermore, arrest may be affected with or without a warrant of arrest. In the case of the *Government of the Republic of South Africa v Basedo and another* [1995] ZASCA 107, the Supreme Court held that section 49(2) of the Criminal Procedure Act 51 of 1977 should not, and indeed cannot, be regarded as a license for the wanton killing of innocent people, nor can any attempt to extend its operation to cases not falling within its ambit be countenanced.

An arrest is made without a warrant of arrest where there is a reasonable suspicion that the person sought to be arrested has committed an offence or is in the process of committing an offence. In the case of *Ndjebo v The Government of the Republic of Namibia* [2017] NAHCMD 140 it was stated that a reasonable suspicion does not equate to what the peace officer subjectively believed when he made the arrest of an accused person. A reasonable suspicion must be an objective reasonable suspicion. In other words, the question is not about a particular peace officer but rather the conclusion that would possibly be reached by any other peace officer in similar circumstances.

The police officer effecting the arrest has a peremptory responsibility to inform the person whom he or she seeks to arrest of the reasons that necessitate the effect of the arrest. If the arrest emanates from a warrant of arrest, the police officer must hand the copy of the warrant to the person to be arrested (section 39(2) Criminal Procedure Act 57 of 1977). The consequence of an arrest is lawful detention; once arrested, an accused person shall be kept in lawful custody until he or she is lawfully discharged from custody. In effecting such an arrest, it is important that police officers act in an ethical manner.

Accountability is one of the principles of good corporate governance and cannot be divorced from ethics and ethical behavior. As much as it is commonly understood as a principle of corporate governance in the context of company law, it is also critical in the criminal justice system. The law enforcement agencies must be held accountable for their compliance with the legal framework. A mere failure in own's responsibility and duty may lead to poor service delivery and a failure to ensure proper functioning of the criminal justice system. Accountability and compliance should not only relate to the police officers who execute their duties, but the whole law enforcement agency, being the police force in this regard, must exercise accountability (Hubbard, 2019).

Each individual and each unit in the criminal justice system is given a unique mandate and performs a specified function at a given point in time. For example, those working at the charge office are responsible for assisting the members of the public that come and report crimes; an investigator performs an investigation on a particular crime that was alleged to have been committed; and the station commander exercises control and responsibility over his or her station. It is important that all these office-bearers take complete responsibility for their offices and perform their tasks with distinction.

Compliance is another important principle that is commonly associated with corporate governance. Compliance is key in any structure or organization. It refers to the conduct of adhering to the laws and policies established in a particular department or sector and which policies or laws are required in the execution of one's duty or function. In order to ensure proper compliance, it is important to develop detailed and concise set of rules, whether in the form of laws, regulations, or policies. Second, it is prime that supervisors and those in command oversee the functions performed by their juniors to ensure that there is proper compliance with what is required. For example, in the police force, a sergeant should oversee the work of a constable, while a warrant officer must oversee the work of the sergeant to ensure proper functioning and effective execution of duties. In other words, a police officer must comply with the law that empowers him or her to effect arrest, and secondly, he or she must comply with the procedures set out for effecting such an arrest.

Investigation and Prosecution

The arrest and detention of an accused person are followed by an investigation and prosecution to prove the innocence or guilt of such a person. The primary purpose of an investigation is to gather all evidence that is used during the prosecution stage. This evidence will assist the adjudicating officer to arrive at a well-informed conclusion regarding the innocence or guilt of the accused person. The date on which the crime was committed, the persons involved in the commission of the crime, the objects used, and the persons that witnessed the commission of the crime are aspects that are considered during the investigation stage. Once the investigating officer has completed his or her investigations, he delivers a file to the prosecutor to conduct the prosecution in terms of the law. The office of the Prosecutor-General is established through the constitutional mandate. Article 88 of the Constitution therefore provides that:

> (1) There shall be a Prosecutor-General appointed by the President on the recommendation of the Judicial Service Commission . . . (2) The powers and functions of the Prosecutor-General shall be: (a) to prosecute, subject to the provisions of this Constitution, in the name of the Republic of Namibia in criminal proceedings; (b) to prosecute and defend appeals in criminal proceedings in the High Court and the Supreme Court; (c) to perform all functions relating to the exercise of such powers.

Apart from the Prosecutor-General other legal officers are appointed under the Prosecutor-General, and their mandate is also derived from the Constitution, in particular to conduct criminal proceedings in any court upon delegated authority by the prosecutor-general. In addition, "(d) to delegate to other officials, subject to his or her control and direction, authority to conduct criminal proceedings in any Court; and (e) to perform all such other functions as may be assigned to him or her in terms of any other law."

Furthermore, section 2 of the Criminal Procedure Act 51 of 1977, vests the authority to prosecute in the State. Thus, a public prosecutor who is employed by the state prosecutes an offense. In the prosecution of an offense, a prosecutor must conduct such prosecution in an ethical manner. There have been instances where public prosecutors have been alleged of helping themselves with witness fees. Witness fees are money set aside by the courts to cover for witnesses traveling from one town to the next to attend court for the purpose of testifying. It is unethical of a prosecutor to take such funds for his or her own use, as it amounts to theft and/or corruption. Such a type of conduct brings the prosecutorial department of the Ministry of Justice into disrepute. In other instances, unethical conduct presents itself in prosecution, where a prosecution is paid money by the accused person in order not to prosecute the offense alleged to have been committed. Again, this is unethical and may even prevent justice from prevailing.

The legal profession generally and the office of a prosecutor in general demand that a prosecutor must be ethical in conducting his or her duties. Oftentimes, allegations are levelled against prosecutors to the effect that they receive bribes, and based on this, they do not conduct prosecutions properly, which results in victims of crimes being denied justice. Although this remains an allegation and may even be unfounded in many instances, if it happens that bribery is actually taking place in the prosecution of crimes, this would have negative and severe consequences, such as the punishing of innocent persons and/or acquitting guilty persons.

In addition to public prosecutions, the Criminal Procedure Act 51 of 1977 provides for private prosecution. Section 5 of the Act provides that:

> Presiding judicial officer may in certain circumstances appoint prosecutor. (1) If the person delegated or appointed to conduct a prosecution in criminal

> proceedings in any court is for any reason unable to discharge that function, or if no such person has been delegated or appointed, the judge or judicial officer presiding at such criminal proceedings may, in writing under his hand, designate any competent person to conduct such prosecution in particular criminal proceedings or in all criminal proceedings on any particular day. (2) A person designated under subsection (1) shall in respect of the exercise of his powers and the discharge of his functions be subject to the control and directions of the attorney-general concerned.

The purpose of private prosecution is to prevent undue delays in the prosecution of crimes and finalization of cases. Public prosecution may be overburdened with high volumes of case load and therefore may not be able to finalize cases in a speedy manner. This may sometimes result in undue delays for accused persons awaiting trial. Thus, private prosecution may aid in this regard.

The Functions of the Court: A General Perspective

The judiciary is one of the three branches of government and primarily assists with performing the functions of checks and balances of the activities of the other two branches of government, i.e., the executive and the legislature. In Namibia the judiciary comprises of the courts, and thus the judicial power is vested in the Supreme Court, the High Court and the Lower Courts of Namibia. The courts are independent and are subject only to the Constitution and the law as contemplated in article 78(3) of the Constitution. This means that no other branch of government or any other person may influence the functioning of the courts or the decisions of presiding officers. The presiding officers thus deliver the judgments without fear or favor. A magistrate or judge occupies a noble office as he or she is vested with the responsibility of upholding the constitution and the law, and therefore the conduct of a judge or magistrate both on the bench and in his or her private dealings should be honorable and highly ethical. From time to time, there are allegations of Magistrates not acting in an ethical manner.

Although the judiciary has always been independent in terms of the Constitution, its independence was further solidified by the enactment of the Judiciary Act 11 of 2015. According to its preamble, the Act was enacted to strengthen the independence of the judiciary in line with Article 78(5) of the Namibian Constitution and, among others, to provide for the administrative and financial matters of the Office of the Judiciary; and to provide for connected or incidental matters. Independence of the judiciary is a well-celebrated move in many jurisdictions, including Namibia. When judiciary is independent from the branches of government, the public seems to have more confidence in its activities, as they feel that judiciary is now free from pressure and control from the government. Thus, the decisions of judges and magistrates may now be viewed as independent and without fear or favor. However, this independence must be treated with care. Although the judiciary is independent, its total detachment from the ministry of justice is not advisable. For political reasons and also for the proper functioning of the courts, it is advisable for the judiciary and the Ministry of Justice to maintain a good working relationship. In Namibia, the Ministry of Justice is headed by the minister, while judiciary is headed by the chief justice. The two office bearers perform different tasks, but work toward the same objective: ensuring justice and upholding the Constitution and the law. It is because of this very reason that these two offices must work independently but "together."

Judges are one of the most important stakeholders in the criminal justice system, and they play the role of detached umpire in Namibia. A judge should not only be well versed with the law, but he must always strive to act fairly and impartially. These are the legal ethics that come with the profession. Judicial professional ethics serve the dual purpose of guiding judges when making their decisions in court, and it also makes the public aware of what to expect from judges (Ferrel, 2012). A practical example can be found in the case where a judge is impartial and is acting biased toward someone because of their skin color or even to favor his or her friends. When it comes to equality, presiding officers are expected to treat all persons in legal proceedings equally and with dignity (Ethical Judicial Conduct). The right to equality is a constitutional right, and a judicial officer who fails to respect and uphold this right not only act unethically but also violates the law.

Another equally important principle of good ethical conduct is competence and diligence. Persons in the criminal justice system are required to perform their duties in a competent and diligent manner. Presiding officers, for example, are expected to deliver judgments without unreasonable delay (Ethical Judicia Conduct). Competence boils down to knowing the content of the law and applying it. Limited knowledge on a specific subject matter, for example, may cause a presiding officer to commit an error of the law, leading to wrong judgments. Another important principle of ethics required of a presiding officer is integrity. Integrity refers to honor. All persons holding office as a judicial officer must understand that they hold an honorable office and conduct themselves in a manner that suits such an office.

In the case of *Visagie v Government of the Republic of Namibia,* [2018] NASC 411, it was stated that mala fides, fraud, and malice constitute a perversion of justice and amount to a deliberate abuse of the exalted judicial office. The court went on to state that an example of this could be found in taking a bribe to benefit one litigant to the prejudice of another or using the judicial office to settle a score with an opponent.

The Court's Function: Excerpts on Sentencing

The court, particularly the presiding officer, has a huge responsibility for deciding the fate of the convicted person. It is important that the presiding officers properly apply their minds when performing the function of sentencing. In the case of *S v Rabie* 1975 (4) SA 855(A) the court held that "punishment must fit the criminal, the crime as well as the interests of society, and must be blended with mercy or compassion." The seriousness of the offense will determine the severity of punishment imposed on the convicted individual. The lighter the offense, the lighter the punishment is more likely to be. However, this is not the only factor to be considered. Other factors include aspects as to whether the accused is the first-time offender or not and whether it would be in the best interest of society that the accused person should be taken out of society for retributive purposes.

Role of Legal Practitioners

Most often, the writings on the criminal justice system seem to exclude legal practitioners. Although *stricto sensu* legal practitioners do not directly fall within the criminal justice system, their duties place them to form indirectly in the criminal justice system. Attorneys are tasked with the difficult task of representing their clients in the best possible way, and the focus is not only on winning the case. Generally, there shouldn't be any expectation for attorneys to have to act unethically or against the morals of society in the name of winning the case. They need to follow the written laws and practices (spirit or letter of the law). A practical example is that of the so-called "rogue" prosecutor who purposefully adopts unethical tactics, such as concealing exculpatory material as defined in *Brady v Maryland*, 373 U.S. 83 (1963), instead of turning it over to the defense as required by due process and ethical rules.

In the case of *Cape Society v Vorster* 1949 (3) SA 421 (*C*), it was held that a legal practitioner is an agent of his or her client, and the legal practitioner represents the client; secondly, a legal practitioner is an officer of the court and therefore is under an obligation to assist the court in the administration of justice. In the case of *State v Baleka and Other*s (4) 1988 (4) SA 688 (T) at 705E-F, the court held that "the administration of justice is founded upon the preservation of the dignity of the courts and that the legal practitioner has the duty to assist the court in upholding it. Although legal practitioners are agents of their clients their duty toward the court overrides their obligation toward their client."

Because of the role legal practitioners play in the administration of justice, it is important that their conduct is ethical and professional. Any conduct of a legal practitioner that falls short of what is legally, ethically, and professionally expected hampers a fair administration of justice and brings the entire criminal justice system into disrepute. The Legal Practitioners Act, 15 of 1995, sets out various conducts that are regarded as dishonorable and fall short of the ethical conduct of a legal practitioner. Section 33 of the Act Legal Practitioner 15 of 1995 provides that it is unethical for a legal practitioner to willfully mislead the court or tribunal or allow it to be misled. It is also dishonorable for a legal practitioner to mislead his or her client in any respect material to a client. Again, this boils down to how the conduct of a legal practitioner may hamper the criminal justice system. The courts, which are functionaries of the criminal justice system, rely on legal practitioners as officers of the court to aid with a fair administration of justice. If these officers of the court make themselves guilty of dishonorable conduct and unethical behavior, justice will never be served, and providing justice is the core aim of the criminal justice system.

In terms of the law, the Law Society of Namibia has been established to deal with all aspects that relate to the functions of legal practitioners. Thus, all persons admitted to practice law in Namibia form part of the Law Society. Once a legal practitioner misbehaves, that is dealt with in accordance with the law. In terms of rule 22(2) of the rules of the Law Society, the Legal Ethics and Investigatory Committee is responsible for advising the Law Society Council on all matters of ethics in the practice of law. As such, the Committee has the powers to investigate the conduct of any member that, in their opinion, may require disciplinary action against and advise the Council of their findings.

In Namibia, various legal practitioners have been subjected to disciplinary conduct as a result of the conduct. The notion that "no one is above the law" equally holds true for legal practitioners, and therefore it is crucial for them to conduct themselves in a professional and ethical manner. The existence of the Law Society and, in particular, the Ethics Committee as well as evidence of disciplinary actions taken against legal practitioners who committed ethical wrongs indicate the seriousness with which unethical conduct is being combated in Namibia. However, the question still remains: is it enough, or is there something that can still be done?

A QUESTION ON DELAY IN JUSTICE

On November 18, 2005, the Namibian Newspaper reported that "manpower shortages, tardy Police investigations and not enough money to employ more staff have all been cited as the reasons for the wheels of justice turning so slowly in Namibia" (Namibian Newspaper; 18 November 2005). In January 2018, the same newspaper again reported that the organization (police force) does not have enough resources (Namibian Newspaper; 17 January 2020).

The shortage of resources (funds) means that the police force cannot recruit new personnel so as to cut costs associated with the wage bill (Namibian Newspaper; 17 January 2020). Cutting costs is essential, as the government is required to promote and practice sustainable development and balance its responsibilities across all sectors of society. However, what does cutting costs in the police sector mean for the society at large? Reported crimes cannot be investigated on time because there is either a lack of police personnel to perform this task or a lack of vehicles that can travel to the crime scene timeously.

In certain cases, police officers, although on the ground, may not have the necessary resources and training to carry out investigations (Namibian Newspaper, November 18, 2005). Although all police officers receive basic training upon becoming a police officer, not all of them go through continuous development. The attitude of officials in the police department toward their work and the society has sequences for the entire criminal justice system. If police officers are negligent in the performance of their duties, this may break the link, and justice will either not be served or will be delayed. Thus, a proper attitude of police officers toward their duties and the society is a crucial factor in guaranteeing effective governance. When it comes to the functions of the court, there are key role players such as the presiding officers, prosecutors, interpreters, witnesses, and court orderly. When it comes to state witnesses, witness fees need to be paid and if the government does not have funds to pay for witness fees, cases cannot be finalized timeously and effectively. In the words of the Chief Justice, "If there are no funds to pay witness fees, no criminal trial can take place," he said. That is a reason for much of the delay in the finalization of criminal trials in our courts (18 November 2005).

ENSURING ETHICS IN THE CRIMINAL JUSTICE SYSTEM

Various stakeholders play a crucial role in ensuring that proper administrative justice takes place in the criminal justice system. If any of the stakeholders fail in their thirst to inculcate the true meaning of ethics and ethical behavior into their subjects, the whole criminal justice system will collapse.

The Role Played by a Law School

Whether as a legal practitioner, a prosecutor, or a magistrate, people practicing in the criminal justice system are expected by law and society to act in an ethical manner. There is nothing wrong with expecting one to conduct himself or herself in an ethical manner, but the question that we often forget to ask is, whose responsibility it is to teach one to be ethical? The Bachelor of Laws (LLB) degree or other equivalent degree taught in a School or Faculty of Law is normally designed in such a way as to provide law students with the theoretical aspects of the law on one hand and practical application of the law on the other. One of the commonly found modules in most law curricula is professional ethics. It is believed that the purpose of this course is to teach students ethics, ethical conduct, and how to deal with clients while managing the client's files properly. A failure to lay a proper foundation with regard to teaching and training law students on how to behave and conduct themselves in an ethical manner may be very disastrous.

In the Namibia context, the aforementioned LLB program has been running for some time now after the Faculty of Law (now known as the School of Law) was established in the 1990s. The faculty has produced a number of law graduates, many of whom now plays a crucial role in the criminal justice system. Though an individual's character is somewhere dependent on his or her personal choices and way of life, somehow the training and teaching that one receives contribute to how one conducts himself or herself in a professional and personal life. The question that one then asks is whether the faculty of law has been doing a proper job of properly training its law students to ensure that they produce well-rounded and highly ethical graduates. Can law graduates from the University of Namibia uphold ethics, or will they comprise good ethical conduct? If, for example, a University of Namibia law graduate becomes a magistrate, will he or she make himself or herself guilty of misconduct by failing to observe his or her oath of office? If a law graduate becomes an admitted legal practitioner, will he or she be able to act honestly, be transparent, and act in the best interests of his or her client? Of course, failing to do so will invite severe consequences for the client, in that the client interests may not be properly protected.

The mishaps experienced in the criminal justice system can partially be prevented if the LLB curricula are properly developed to ensure that students are properly taught ethics and properly trained to function in the criminal justice system. This means that students must be acquainted with aspects of the criminal justice system from early days. It is crucial for anyone aspiring to become a criminal lawyer, a judge in the criminal stream or practicing criminal lawyer to fully appreciate both procedural aspects of criminal law and procedure and the substantive elements of criminal law and procedure. The mere fact that the media reports misconduct committed by those in practice whether public or private, indicates that more needs to be done to ensure that when one is admitted to an office of legal professional, he or she observes the oath he or she has taken. Although training legal professionals is the first step toward the practice of law, there are many other factors involved in upholding principles of ethics. A properly trained individual may also change his or her ways in the practice of law. However, this should not prevent academics in law schools from properly training law students.

Good Governance

Corporate governance, used broadly, refers to the procedures, norms, regulations, and institutions that set the direction for how organizations and corporations behave, manage, and oversee their activities. It works to accomplish the organization's objectives and oversees ties with stakeholders. (Khan, 2011, pp. 1–5). Studying this definition makes it clear that in order to have a properly running organization, it is imperative to implement good corporate governance principles within one's organization.

Ethical leadership is the first principle of corporate governance as contained in King II, and as such, ethics and values are vital in any area of leadership (Awarab, 2017, pp. 213–230). In order to ensure good governance, it is thus important for all persons in the criminal justice system to conduct their activities in an ethical manner. All ethical conduct is necessary for everyone; it is more important for those in leadership. Leaders of any organization take decisions and give directives on a daily basis, and thus it is important for such persons to ensure that their conduct and decisions do not conflict with the notion of ethics.

It is essential for those in leadership to hold their subordinates accountable for their actions. For example, in Magistracy, the chief magistrate is the administrative head of Magistracy. It is very crucial for the office of the chief magistrate to ensure that good governance structures are put in place and all those directly accountable to the office of the chief magistrate adhere to such structures and implement them.

In prosecution, it is equally important for the prosecutor-general to ensure that the governance structures that have been established work well in carrying out the mandate of the office. Control prosecutors, for example, must ensure that those over whom they exercise authority adhere to the law and standing rules on procedure.

Continuous Training

Continuous training and skill development is very crucial in any organization. All persons employed in the criminal justice system must undergo continuous training and development to enhance their knowledge and skills. It is therefore crucial for the human resources departments to assess their performance individually and collectively to determine the training needs of persons and offices in the criminal justice system. This chapter does not dispute the fact that training is taking place in various sectors of the criminal justice system.

However, due to the problems experienced in the criminal justice system, for example, the undue delay in the finalization of investigations or a long period it takes before a trial is finalized, it is important that continuous skill development become mandatory.

The Magistracy, for example, hosted a Magistrates workshop. One such training was the Magistrates workshop that was held in 2020, where Magistrates from all regions of Namibia gathered in Windhoek on the theme of "Changing the face of Magistracy: Balancing Independence and Accountability." Training of such nature is very crucial as it refreshes Magistrates on their mandate and the oath that they have taken. It could be beneficial to the Magistracy if a training of this nature takes place annually. Apart from annual training, it is crucial to have workshops where Magistrates can, for example, share ideas and experiences and do peer teaching on subjects that affects their offices as well as Magistracy as a whole. As Magistracy is a noble sector of judiciary, training on ethics should become a must, as ethical behavior is crucial in Magistracy. Apart from the Magistracy, other sectors of the criminal justice sector should introduce and continuously conduct training and skills development programs to further equip persons for office. Such training should revolve around ethics and ethical conduct.

POST-COVID-19 IMPLICATIONS

There is no adequate statistical data that was captured regarding the post-COVID-19 operations in the criminal justice system. However, it is very much possible that the factors that comprise ethics and ethical behavior during COVID-19 will no longer affect operations in the criminal justice system. One factor that will mostly persist to affect service delivery in the criminal justice system is a lack of funds. Before COVID-19, the government did not have enough finances to recruit sufficient personnel to ensure efficient and effective service delivery. During COVID-19, the government spent millions on curbing the spread of COVID-19 and also taking care of its citizens, especially the less privileged and unemployed. Thus, funds that could be used to ensure good service delivery were channeled to other activities during COVID-19, and it will take time to normalize the government budget and ensure that funds are channeled to where there is a need in the criminal justice system.

CONCLUDING REMARKS AND RECOMMENDATIONS

Ethics and ethical behavior should be inculcated at a very young age of an individual. Primarily, law school should include ethical programs at a university level that provide law students with the know-how on proper ethical conduct. Teaching law students' theoretical aspects of the law without combining them with the proper practice of the law is not enough. Although in the Namibian context, it is clear that the Legal Aid and Professional Ethics module ought to provide students with thorough understanding of proper legal and ethical conduct. However, seeing the end product, whether as a legal practitioner, magistrate, or public prosecutor, one cannot help but ask the question as to whether the LLB curriculum through the Legal Aid and Professional Ethics modules provides the students with the required skills and training that will aid them in good ethical conduct.

Another opportunity where candidates can be taught professional ethics is at the justice training center in the module of Professional Ethics. Again, there is a need to revisit the JTC curriculum to ensure that the Professional Ethics module enhances the knowledge of candidates on professional and ethical conduct. In the case of courts and judicial officers, and in order to prevent the backlog of cases, it is important for the office of the judiciary to employ enough judicial officers to deal with cases timeously. Furthermore, in the adjudication of cases, although each case is to be dealt with on its own merits, it is important to ensure that proper and standard procedures are followed. A classic example of a wrongdoing often committed by Magistrates is the failure to follow proper procedure with regard to pleas in terms of section 112 and section 115.

In terms of the regulations, there is a requirement that review judgments from the Magistrates Courts must be sent to the High Court for review. It is crucial that mechanisms are put in place to ensure that review judgments reach the High Court. This can be a way in which Magistrate's whole judgments are not in line can be identified for training and skill development. Chief Magistrate should continuously have executive meeting with divisional magistrates. This type of meetings would serve two purposes. One leg is for the Chief Magistrate to understand possible problems that magistrates are facing, while the second leg is to provide advice and guidance. Similarly, the director and the chairperson of the law society should have quarterly meetings with all admitted legal practitioners to provide guidance and advise on ethical conduct and ethical leadership.

All stakeholders in the criminal justice system need to play an active role to ensure the establishment and maintaining high standards in the criminal justice system.

Owners of law firms and those in the law practice should understand that, though money is important, upholding the practice of the law is important. In order to win public trust and confidence, all key stakeholders in the criminal justice system must perform their task diligently. The first step toward executing the mandate effectively starts with knowing what is expected.

Most organs in the criminal justice system are creatures of statute and thus derive their powers from the statute. It is imperative that those involved in the criminal justice system acquaint themselves with the provisions of the statute, more so to find out what their powers and duties are. The government can implement mandatory workshops targeting certain individuals with the aim of introducing and reminding functionaries in the criminal justice system about their rights and duties.

The police sector of the criminal justice system normally organizes police training, which is attended by police officers, and upon completion, the latter receives a completion certificate. This is a good gesture in keeping the police officers well-informed with regard to the law. However, this gesture can be more effective and will yield better results if the Ministry of Home Affairs, Immigration, and Safety and Security partners with institutions of higher level and makes it mandatory for police officers to undergo courses to enhance the latter's knowledge and keep them abreast of the law. Effective leadership is very crucial in every sector. Thus, it is important that those in leadership of criminal justice system, which are the commanders, are well knowledgeable in the area of good corporate governance. When they make decisions, they must take the corporate governance principles into consideration as their decisions may have a long-term effect and bearing on the criminal justice system.

REFERENCES

Awarab, M. "Corporate Governance and Municipalities: Are the King III Principles Exportable to Local Government in Namibia?" in *The Law Reform and Development Commission of Namibia at 25: A Quarter Century of Social Carpentry*, edited by Dunia Zongwe and Yvonne Dausab (2017). Ministry of Justice, Law Reform and Development Commission.

Belshaw, S.H., Johnstone, P., & Deboer, L. *Ethics in the Criminal Justice System*. 2nd ed. Kendall Hunt Publisher (2020). 978-1-4652-7606-3

Cape Society v Vorster 1949 (3) SA 421 (C).

Criminal Procedure Act 51 of 1977.

Ferrell, C. Ethics and Professionalism: No Lying, Cheating or Stealing. *The Police Chief* (2012).

Holmes, R. *Basic Moral Philosophy* (4th ed.). Belmont, CA: Wadsworth (1998).

Khan, H. International Proceedings of Economics Development and Research IPEDR Vol. 25 (2011), pp. 1–5.

Legal Practitioners Act 15 of 1995.

Namibian Constitution.

Namibian Newspaper: Criminal Justice System Overstretched (18 November 2015).

Namibian Newspaper: Lack of Resources Affecting Police Services (17 January 2017).

Newham, G. "Why Police Leadership Matters." *SA Crime Quarterly* Vol. 53, No. 53 (2015), pp. 39–48.
Nomfundo Manyathi-Jele. "Can Ethics Be Taught?." *De Rebus*, No. 540 (2014), pp. 8–11.
Pieter Petrus Visagie v Government of the Republic of Namibia and Others [2018] NASC 411.
Police Act 19 of 1990.
S v Rabie 1975 (4) SA 855(A).
Shakil, M. "Criminal Justice System: Social Work and Corrections." *International Journal of Society and Humanities* Vol. 6, No. 1 (2015). ISSN-2319-2070.
Singer, P. *How Are We to Live? Ethics in an Age of Self-Interest.* Amherst, NY: Prometheus Books (1995).
State v Baleka and Others (4) 1988 (4) SA 688 (T) at 705E-F.
The Government of the Republic of South Africa v Basedo and another [1995] ZASCA 107.
Ushinge v Government of the Republic of Namibia (HC-MD-CIV-ACT-DEL-2018/00243) [2020] NAHCMD 341 (7 August 2020).

Chapter 3

Use of Force during COVID-19 Pandemic

A South African Perspective

Malematja Stanley and Udochu Eke

INTRODUCTION

The COVID-19 pandemic placed the world under unique and unprecedented times. Countries across the globe implemented national lockdowns in efforts to curb its spread, while scientists worked tirelessly to find a vaccine. Lockdowns led to the limitation of certain fundamental human rights, such as the right to freedom of movement and peaceful assembly. Furthermore, states amplified their security by deploying and centralizing law enforcement agencies to enforce restrictions put in place to curb COVID-19. In South Africa, drastic measures were taken; economic activities were halted, and certain human rights were limited for the duration of the lockdown, which commenced on March 26, 2020. After the declaration of the national state of disaster, the minister of cooperative governance and traditional affairs promulgated the regulations in terms of section 27(2) of the Disaster Management Act 57 of 2002. The regulations were commonly known as the "lockdown regulations" and will be discussed later in this chapter.

Without the availability of a cure or vaccine for the virus, people were advised and urged to avoid unnecessary movements and maintain social distancing when they were in public spaces. Other safety measures included the wearing of face masks. In South Africa, the measures introduced by the government were meant to flatten the curve and allow the medical sector to prepare the fight against the virus. The South African government went as far as deploying the South African National Defense Force (SANDF) to assist the South Africa Police Services (SAPS) to implement the lockdown regulations, which involved controlling and/or prohibiting certain movements by civilians. According to section 33(1)(a) – (i) of the Disaster Management Act 2002 (2002, May 28), exceptions on movement of people were made, including going to school, going to places of employment, buying essential goods or essential obtaining services, and the transportation of mortal remains. The enforcement of the lockdown regulations resulted in several human rights violations. The state security forces had on several occasions implemented unlawful, cruel, and dehumanizing punishment on those alleged to have contravened the lockdown regulations. Over five people died in the hands of state security forces respectively during the implementation of the lockdown regulations (Heywood, 2020). Others have been met with dehumanizing and unlawful punishment, including smacking, kicking, push-ups, and being made to roll on the ground.

This chapter critically analyzes the use of force by state security forces in the process of enforcing the lockdown regulations. The chapter also considers cases of use of force reported by the media. Moreover, the chapter gives an overview of the existing legal framework that regulates the use of force. In essence, it is contended that law enforcement agencies often use unreasonably disproportionate and deadly force. This contention is supported by the analysis of the judgment of the *Khosa Mpepu & Others v Minister of Defence and Military Veteran & Others* 21512/2020, dealt with later in the chapter.

SYNOPSIS OF THE USE OF FORCE IN SOUTH AFRICA

Issues pertaining to the manner of policing in South Africa date back to the apartheid era, where policing was based on racial and oppressive laws sought to suppress the black majority of the country. The structure of the then-police unit was not only exemplified by the use of excessive and deadly force. The deployment structure was also problematic; black policers were exposed to daily violence while white police officers were settled in headquarters in Pretoria (Brogden, 1994, 26). The police unit of South Africa is well known for its gun-brazen attitude and its non-hesitant nature to shoot to kill unarmed civilians (Brogden, 1994, 19). At the advent of the dawn of democracy, the South African Police was transformed to South African Police Service and this was to dismantle the military police force nature of the unit and to bring a policing unit that, inter alia, maintains law and order and prevents crime.

The essential change for the police was also to enable accountability in cases of police brutality and criminality. As part of the post-apartheid reform of the South African Police, the government established the Independent Police Investigative Directorate (IPID). The mission of IPID is to ensure independent oversight over the South African Police Service (SAPS) and the Municipal Police Services (MPS), and to conduct independent and impartial investigations of identified criminal offences allegedly committed by members of the SAPS and the MPS, and make appropriate recommendations. (Independent Police Investigative Directorate, 2013, 3)

Despite a clear mandate, IPID's handling of cases is appalling, investigations are prematurely closed, and only few cases are referred to the National Prosecution Authority for prosecution (Knoetze, 2019). Such incomplexity by IPID fails victims of police brutality as well as eroding the justice system and therefore exacerbating police brutality. Furthermore, it aids and abets the police to commit criminal offenses with impunity.

State security forces are inclined to use lethal force when implementing the law in the country. They use firearms to disperse crowds during gatherings or to maintain law and order during a civil unrest (Haysom, 1987, 5). When force is used, the violation of fundamental rights is inevitable predominately, the violation of the right to human dignity and the right to life. The right to life is a constitutionally guaranteed right enshrined in section 11 of the Constitution of South Africa, 1996. The state has duty to ensure the protection of this right from any arbitrary deprivation. The right to life is arguably the most important human right because once one is deprived of this right, the other rights become moot. Notwithstanding that, there are circumstances that justify the legal use of lethal force. This includes a situation in which a police officer is under an obligation to protect another person or property or him/herself (*R v Brits* 1949 (3) SA 293 at 304). The enforcement of the lockdown regulations seldom includes a situation where a state security officer finds him/herself having to protect a person from an imminent lethal attack, which would justify the use of lethal force.

Despite the latter assertion, in less than two months since the commencement of the national lockdown, the South African Military Ombud Office received 28 complaints, and at least 15 out of the 28 complaints were from the public alleging excessive use of force by the members of SANDF during patrols (Good Governance Africa, 2020). On the other hand, the IPID recorded 39 complaints against police misconduct and acts of *ultra vires* in the enforcement of the lockdown regulations (Gumede, 2020). When the military was deployed to assist the police to enforce the lockdown regulations, people questioned the deployment and raised issues of foreseeable human rights violations. Between March 23 and 25, 2020, the minister of defense was interviewed on a popular radio station (Talk Radio 702), and the minister assured the public that the soldiers were deployed to assist the police to enforce the law in line with the Constitution. The assurance was essentially that no human rights will be violated, not at least through the use of excessive force. However, the direct opposite of what the Minister assured occurred. On April 11, 2020, four members of SANDF fatally assaulted a man in Alexandra township after it was alleged that he disobeyed the orders from two female members of SANDF (*Khosa Mpepu & Others v Minister of Defence and Military Veteran & Others* 21512/2020).

In response to the fatal attack on the unarmed man who posed no threat to the soldiers, the Minister of Defense said, "we hang our head in shame" (Gumede, 2020). It shall be noted that to hang one's head in shame is not equivalent to taking accountability or action against the unlawful conduct of the soldiers. After incidents of police brutality, it is common for leaders to publicly denounce the incidents and promise punishment against the police but in reality, such promises are distasteful (Foster & Luyt, 1986, 277). State security is seldom held accountable for police brutality and/ or murder (Kings, 2013). It is actually concerning that 26 years into democracy, our state security forces still conduct itself in a manner that depicts no knowledge of human rights or the respect thereof (Gumede, 2020). To a certain extent, the vile behavior by members of the defense force during the pandemic is not surprising because the National Defense Force General publicly said, "when we come in, we skop and donder" (an Afrikaans phrase and when directly translated to English, it means "kick and assault or harm"). In a subsequent media briefing, the president of the Republic said, "this is not the time to skop and donder." Despite the president's announcement, a political leader belonging to the ruling party, the African National Congress, was recorded encouraging soldiers to "skop and donder" those who transgressed the lockdown regulations (Head, 2020). It is such statements by political leaders and people in higher positions in public offices that exacerbate police and/or military brutality. Police and/or military brutality translates to ill-treatment or torture.

INTERNATIONAL AND REGIONAL LEGAL MECHANISMS ON THE USE OF FORCE

South Africa is a party state to several international instruments of the United Nations (UN) and the African Union (AU) on the use of force by state security forces to the extent that they perform law enforcement functions. By signing and ratifying the United Nations Convention Against Torture and other Cruel, Inhumane and Degrading Treatment of Punishment 1984 (UNCAT), South Africa aimed to strengthen its efforts and measures to prevent torture, cruel, inhuman, and degrading treatment or punishment. Furthermore, the ratification of the instrument galvanizes the exposing of places of detention to public scrutiny and makes sure that the entire system in which police, security, and intelligence officials operate is more transparent and accountable to external monitoring. In 2006, South Africa signed the Optional Protocol to the United Nations Convention Against Torture (the Protocol). Article 1 of the convention defines torture as

> any act by which severe pain or suffering, whether physical or mental, is intentionally inflicted on a person for such purposes as obtaining from him or a third person information or a confession, punishing him for an act he or a third person has committed or is suspected of having committed, or intimidating or coercing him or a third person, or for any reason based on discrimination of any kind, when such pain or suffering is inflicted by or at the instigation of or with the consent or acquiescence of a public official or other person acting in an official capacity.

Article 5 of the Universal Declaration of Human Rights, 1948 states that, "no one shall be subjected to torture or to cruel, inhumane, or degrading treatment or punishment." Certain articles of this declaration that can be suspended when strictly necessary for "the life of a nation." However, Article 5 is not one of them. A global pandemic can never be a justification for subjecting people to torture, cruel, inhumane, or degrading punishment or treatment.

The right to freedom from torture and other dehumanizing treatment is also recognized in the African Charter on Human and Peoples' Rights 1996 (ACHPR). According to Article 5 of the ACHPR, "All forms of exploitation and degradation of man particularly [. . .] torture, cruel, inhuman or degrading punishment and treatment shall be prohibited." The excessive use of force is prohibited under these provisions. According to Article 7 of the International Covenant on Civil and Political Right (ICCPR), "No one shall be subjected to torture or to cruel, inhuman or degrading treatment or punishment." Articles 4 and 16 of UNCAT provide an akin protection. When the SANDF personnel patrolled the township streets in South Africa, people were met with the most degrading punishment when found roaming the streets. They were kicked, smacked, made to do exercises, and forced to roll in dirty, muddy water. This type of inhumane punishment serves no other legitimate purpose but the infliction of pain or suffering. Article 4.1 of the UNCAT requires state party parties to criminalize any act of torture. This implies that state security involved in acts of unreasonable and disproportionate use of force and torture shall be tried by the criminal justice system of the country, and if found guilty, then suitable punishment shall follow. The use of force is guided by two principles: the principle of proportionality and the principle of minimum force (Haysom, 1987, 8). The principle of minimum force requires state security to use lethal force as a measure of last resort, and the proportionality principle requires force to be proportionate to the legitimate end result, for example, arrest or detention (Haysom, 1987, 8).

ASPECTS OF THE USE OF FORCE AND POLICE BRUTALITY: DOMESTIC LAW AND POLICY

South Africa is hailed for having the most progressive Constitution in the world, with a comprehensive Bill of Rights. According to section 12(1) of the Constitution

> everyone has the right to freedom and security of the person, which includes the right- (a) not to be deprived of the freedom arbitrarily or without justice; (b) not to be detained without fair trial; (c) to be free from all forms of violence from either public or private sources; (d) not to be tortured in any way and; (e) not to be treated or punished in a cruel, inhumane or degrading way.

The provision at hand is vivid on the freedom and security of a person, and it protects individuals against ill-treatment either by the state or private persons. When law enforcement officers are executing their duties, it is pivotal that they abide by the Constitution, especially in relation to the respect and protection of fundamental human rights. Despite the existence of this crystal-clear constitutional provision, police had already killed three people within five days of the national lockdown (Faull, 2020). Section 205(3) of the Constitution provides that "the objects of the police services are to prevent, combat and investigate crime, to maintain public order, to protect and secure the inhabitants of the Republic and their property, and to enforce the law." It is during the enforcement of the law that the police often violate human rights. The violation of human rights by the police is not akin to the pandemic; there is actually a long history of police brutality in South Africa (Izobo & Abiodun, 2020).

State security is permitted to utilize force only when it is imperative and to the extent required to perform duties. Duties of state security officers involve securing an arrest, and such an arrest is secured for purposes of bringing an accused person before a court of law. Section 37(1)(b) of the Disaster Management Act empowers a law enforcement official to use force appropriate to effect an arrest, and such force must conform to the relevant provisions of the Criminal Procedure Act 51 of 1977 (Criminal Procedure Act). Section 39(1) of the Criminal Procedure Act permits a law enforcer to use force in limited circumstances in order to arrest a person, the force used must be aimed at confining the person who is resting an arrest. Section 49(2) of the Criminal Procedure Act provides that:

> If any arrestor attempts to arrest a suspect and the suspect resists the attempt, or flees, or resists the attempt and flees, when it is clear that an attempt to arrest him or her is being made, and the suspect cannot be arrested without the use of force, the arrestor may, in order to effect the arrest, use such force as may

> be reasonably necessary and proportional in the circumstances to overcome the resistance or to prevent the suspect from fleeing, but, in addition to the requirement that the force must be reasonably necessary and proportional in the circumstances, the arrestor may use deadly force only if- (a) the suspect poses a threat of serious violence to the arrestor or any other person; or (b) the suspect is suspected on reasonable grounds of having committed a crime involving the infliction or threatened infliction of serious bodily harm and there are no other reasonable means of effecting the arrest, whether at that time or later.

According to the abovementioned provision, appropriate and reasonable force may be used to secure an arrest, not to torture or ill-treat a person, as we depicted in numerous videos that surfaced on social media. According to section 6.2.1 of the guidelines for the use of force and torture, a police officer or soldier may not, under no circumstances, arrest a person in order to punish, scare, harass, or teach that person a lesson. The conduct of the soldiers and police did not only violate fundamental human rights but also derailed and eroded the principles of a democratic society. Soldiers and police acted above the law; they punished people for alleged non-compliance with the lockdown regulations. In South Africa, punishment subsequent to the failure to comply with the law rests with the judiciary and not the law enforcement officers. Apart from having a duty to protect people from acts of torture, section 10 of the Prevention of Combating and Torture of Persons Act 13 of 2013 (the Torture Act) obliges the state to promote awareness against the prohibition of torture acts. This implies that state security must be trained in the prevention, prohibition, and combating of acts of torture. Such training also instils public trust toward the state security. In the case of *F v Minister of Safety and Security* 2012 (1) SA 536 CC, the apex court in the land held that the Constitution advocates for the public's trust in the police and that if the police break such trust, it erodes the principles of a democratic and constitutional society. What we have observed during the lockdown was not only unlawful, inhumane, and barbaric acts by the police and soldiers; it is also acts of defying the Constitution, international instruments, and domestic laws and policies.

It is crucial for the reader to understand the context regarding the deployment of the defense force (soldiers) to assist the police to enforce the lockdown regulations. The deployment of the defense force was authorized by the President in terms of section 201(2)(a) of the Constitution and section 18(1) of the Defence Act 42 of 2002 (the Defence Force Act), in cooperation with the police to enforce the lockdown regulations. Together, they were deployed under a joint operation called "Operation Notlela," meaning lock (*Khosa Mpepu & Others v Minister of Defence and Military Veteran & Others,* 2020, p. 17). The deployment of the defense force in such circumstances comes with conditions, such as that the defense force members are subject to the provisions of the South African Police Services Act 68 of 1995 (the SAPS

Act) and the Criminal Procedure Act. Like section 10 of the Torture Act, section 20(1) of the SAPS Act provides for the appropriate training of members of the defense force. The training is crucial because soldiers are trained to use force as opposed to refraining from it. The training is of paramount importance when such military personnel are deployed to enforce laws. The laws such as the Disaster Management Act, which includes the regulation of the movement of people during a state of disaster and not combat against an enemy. Furthermore, the defense force must be guided by a Code of Conduct aimed at re-educating the members to cease from a militarized approach and to one of civilian control without the use of force. Andrew Faull (2020), in his brief article titled "State abuses could match the threat of COVDI-19 itself," posed essential questions such as: "are law enforcers prepared for the nuance of this challenge? What guidelines have they been given? What tools?" (Faull, 2020, p. 3). An attempt at these questions is made through the analysis of the judgment below. Andrew rightfully contends that carrying semi-automatic refiles in the current context is irrelevant; the members of the defense force should have been equipped with food parcels, COVID-19 protective equipment, and pamphlets to distribute to the public (Faull, 2020).

ANALYSIS OF *KHOSA MPEPU AND OTHERS* CASE

In *Khosa Mpepu & Others v Minister of Defence and Military Veteran & Others* 21512/2020, the Applicants approached the High Court to seek relief and a declaratory order in respect of the entitlement to the fundamental right to human dignity (section 10 of the Constitution), the right to life (section 11 of the Constitution), the right not be tortured in any form (section 12(1)(e) of the Constitution) and that the members of SAPS, SANDF, and MPS are bound by the provisions of Prevention and Combating of Torture of Persons Act and the United Nations Convention Against Torture (*Khosa Mpepu & Others v Minister of Defence and Military Veteran & Others* 21512/2020). Furthermore, the Applicants sought relief from the court that the members of SANDF, SAPS, and MPS must adhere to the Constitution, particularly the Bill of Rights, when enforcing the lockdown regulations. Moreover, the members of SANDF, SAPS, and MPS must adhere to the laws regarding minimum and reasonable use of force to perform an official duty. The High Court further ordered the suspension of the members of the SANDF. In addition, the command chain of SAPS, SANDF, and MPS was urged to warn its members that failure to report matters of torture and degrading and inhumane punishment would expose the concerned member to criminal and/or civil claims. The court also ordered the SAPS to promulgate guidelines on the use of minimal, reasonable, and appropriate force, adequate to carry out their official duties. In a constitutional state like South Africa, the latter order shall be a norm and praxis.

The relief was sought after members of the SANDF brutally assaulted a man who later succumbed to the injuries inflicted through torture and inhumane and degrading punishment and treatment. On April 10, 2020, which was "Good Friday," a holiday celebrated by the South African Christian community, a man by the name of Colins Khosa (hereinafter referred to as the deceased) was brutally assaulted and tortured by members of SANDF for consuming alcohol in his yard. The deceased and his brother-in-law were confined to their homes as required by the section 11B(1)(a) of the Disaster Management Act (the lockdown regulations). It is noteworthy that the lockdown regulations prohibited the sale and dispensation of alcohol thereof. On that fateful day, two members of SANDF entered the home of the deceased with sjamboks (a whip made of rubber and plastic) and found the deceased and his brother-in-law in their yard consuming liquor. The members of SANDF accused the deceased and his brother-in-law of violating the lockdown regulations. Such an accusation should have been followed by an arrest, not torture and inhumane punishment.

Subsequent to accusations, the two members of SANDF questioned the deceased about a camping chair and a cup of liquor. All this was happening in the yard of the deceased. The deceased responded and said the law does not prohibit him from consuming liquor in his own yard, a private space. That was his mistake, having knowledge of the relevant law. The members of SANDF then raided the deceased's house, confiscated beer from his fridge, and ordered him to follow them to the street. On their way out, they damaged the deceased's vehicle, and the deceased questioned the vandalism. While in the street, the members of SANDF called for backup and other members of SANDF and Johannesburg Metropolitan Police responded. Three other members of SANDF manhandled the unarmed and compliant, Mr. Khosa. They choked him while pouring beer on top of his head. They proceeded to slam him against a concrete wall, hit him with butt of a machine gun, slapped, kicked, and punched him in the stomach and rib cage. Some community members filmed the brutal incident on their phones, and they were spotted by the soldiers, who demanded that they delete the footage. The community members were loaded into a vehicle by the Johannesburg Metropolitan Police, dropped off kilometers away from their homes, and their phones thrown away in bushes. Other two soldiers proceeded to the house of the deceased, where one of them repeatedly whipped the deceased's wife. After the ordeal, the soldiers and police left. The deceased began to vomit and lost speech and consciousness.

The wife of the deceased called the deceased's brother-in-law, who then contacted the emergency services. Unfortunately, Mr. Khosa was certified dead on arrival. A post-mortem report ruled blunt trauma force to the head and torso as the cause of death. Even the death notice "described cause of death as a blunt force head injury". However, an inquiry by SANDF exonerated the soldiers of the death of Mr. Khosa. It is not shocking because such inquiries are less threatening to its members (Kollapen, 1993, 5). A report filed in the court papers stated that the deceased was not killed by the soldiers. In its feeble defense, the Minister of Defense said the soldiers only smacked the deceased. They went on to say that they smacked him because he disrespected the two female soldiers who questioned him about the beer and camping chair in his yard. The Defense Minister's porous defense weaponized gender inequality; they used the gender of the female soldiers as a justification for the murder of the deceased. To add salt to an open wound, the police ministry issued a statement that it would be appealing the High Court judgment, particularly an order that Minister of Police and Minister of Defense, respectively, must engage in an investigation on the treatment of people whose rights may have been infringed by the SANDF, SAPS, or MPS during the national disaster (Sidimba, 2020).

A CRITICAL ASSESSMENT OF THE USE OF FORCE IN LIGHT OF THE KHOSA JUDGMENT

It is uncontested that the deceased and his brother-in-law were not accused of having committed a crime involving the infliction or threatened infliction of serious bodily harm. If a crime was at all committed, the deceased could have been arrested without torture or harm. It is clear from the facts of the case that the objective of the soldiers was to punish the deceased by inflicting *corpus* pain, which resulted in the death of the deceased. The deceased in the above case died a painful death. The only "crime" he committed was telling the female soldiers that the law prohibits him from purchasing alcohol as opposed to consuming it in his private space. Consequently, he was met with deadly force, torture, and then death. South Africa has a plethora of laws, including the Constitution of 1996, the SAPS Act, and the Criminal Procedure Act, that caution and regulate the use of force by state security. Our police and soldiers disregard the Constitution of this country. Laws and policies are just as good as their implementation. Our leaders lack the will to implement laws, thus allowing police and soldiers to torture and kill people. In response to the death of Mr. Khosa, the Minister of Defense said civilians must not provoke the soldiers, thus blaming Mr. Khosa for his own death. In case at hand, the minister annexed a document titled "Joint-operations Divisional Operational Directive to Charlie Company of 21 South African Infantry Battalion of 30 March 2020" to the court papers.

Charlie Company was deployed to patrol the streets of Alexandra township, the place where Mr. Khosa was killed. The directive of this company was not in line with civilian policing aimed at assisting SAPS; rather, it was characterized by military combat and engagement against antagonist forces. Clearly, the Charlie Company allows the soldiers to use force, which is not aimed at securing an arrest but at punishing a suspect. In an affidavit by the deceased's brother-in-law in the above case, he said that the soldiers took the deceased to the street to "teach him a lesson". When the deceased was punished, he was a mere "suspect". The force that was applied to the deceased was to severely injure and kill him. In answering the questions posed by Andrew and with reference to the Charlie Company, the mission of soldiers deployed in Alexandra township is to punish any person suspected of transgressing the lockdown laws.

The soldiers who killed Mr. Khosa acted with impunity because the leaders seldom hold them accountable for acts of torture and inhumane and degrading punishment. Police at the scene just watched as the soldiers punished Mr. Khosa. It is such acts that allow law enforcement officials to brutalize people. Months succeeding the death of Mr. Khosa, the Minister of Police responded to protests against police brutality and said, "There is no police brutality in society and we should not behave as if police do as they please" (Covid-19 anti-repression working group, 2020, p. 2). On April 22, 2020, the chief of staff of SANDF and the Charlie Company appeared before Parliament's Joint Standing Committee, and when questioned, the Lieutenant General said SANDF does not report to parliamentarians and only takes instructions from the Commander in Chief (*Khosa Mpepu & Others v Minister of Defence and Military Veteran & Others*). Such behavior endorses conduct that continues to undermine the constitutional dispensation and the human rights that come with it. Furthermore, such conduct by state security takes us back to the evil apartheid system, where the police and soldiers punished and killed people with impunity (Mutua, 1997, 71). The use of excessive force is not a problem unique to South Africa, and the lack of accountability by law enforcement appears to be a praxis other parts of the world (Wekili & Leus, 1994, 173). The fact that soldiers can raid the personal space of a civilian and proceed to assault him in front of police says a lot about the type of system in South Africa. The duty of the police and soldiers equally is to protect people, not harm them. If the intention is to arrest, the force used must be limited to that intention. When Mr. Khosa was brutally assaulted, his hands were held to his back, thus an arrest was already carried out. Pouring beer on his head and striking him with the butt of a machine gun was an act of criminality punishable by the law. But the killers of Mr. Khosa still patrol the streets, and the accountability from the Minister of Defense was "hanging her head in shame" (Gumede, 2020).

A COMPARATIVE ANALYSIS OF SOUTH AFRICA AND NAMIBIA

In general, colonialism defined the nature and structure of policing on the African continent (Dessil & Tait, 2011, 1). Consequently, police in the Southern African region have been perceived by the civilian population as brutal and corrupt (Dessil & Tait, 2011, 1). While the Republic of South Africa ratified the UNCAT, the Republic of Namibia acceded to it on November 28, 1994. In efforts to curb the spread of the coronavirus, several countries in the SADC region implemented national lockdowns. Namibia declared a state of emergency in terms of Article 26(1) of its Constitution, 1990. The socioeconomic fabric of South Africa and Namibia is arguably similar in pattern. Many African countries gained independence in the 1960s; Namibia was infiltrated by apartheid South Africa, and the evil regime's laws were used to deny black Namibians socioeconomic and political rights (South African History Online, 2019). The main message regarding minimizing the infection and curbing the spread of the coronavirus is the washing of hands and social distancing.

Both in South Africa and Namibia, water and sanitation remain a dream for the majority of black people (Gawanas, 2020). "In Namibia, law enforcement officials are already subjected to criminal sanction when they use excessive force, both in theory and in practice" (Hubbard, Van Dijcke, Touré, Cooper & Engelbrecht, 2019, 77). There is an undeniable global drive to end police brutality and the disproportional use of force by law enforcement officers. Experts on human rights are concerned about the use of force by police in enforcing lockdown regulations, and it has been found that civilians are subjected to cruel and humiliating punishment (Gonese, Shivamba & Meerkotter, 2020). Like in South Africa, police brutality is a lived reality in Namibia. While the pandemic exposed the deep inequalities in South African society, on the other hand, it magnified police brutality and the disproportionate and unreasonable use of force in Namibia (Namibia Fact Check, 2020). Namibia Fact Check (2020) further reported that on March 3, 2020, David Tuhafeni from Ohangwena Region died after an alleged assault by two police officers. Namibia Fact Check (2020) had an interview with the lawyer of the deceased's family, and it was found that the deceased was assaulted in his home after he questioned an act of police brutality he had witnessed. In a separate incident, Namibia Fact Check (2020) reported that two men were assaulted by the police because they "talked too much".

It is noteworthy that Article 8(2)(b) of the Constitution of the Republic of Namibia guarantees the right of protection against torture and cruel, inhumane, or degrading treatment or punishment. Article 24(3) of the Constitution of the Republic of Namibia makes torture and other ill-treatment non-derogable. However, even with such clear and precise provisions in place, police brutality and excessive use of force remain an issue in the country. This further goes against Article 1 of the Code of Conduct of the Police Officials, which requires the police to respect and uphold the fundamental right to human dignity and maintain and uphold all human rights. Research by African Policing Civilian Oversight Forum (APCOF) found issues in police training in human rights (APCOF, 2012, 14). The fact is that the police in Namibia received training in military tactics, and there has been a struggle to incorporate such police officers into civilian policing (APCOF, 2012, 103). The enforcement of a national lockdown does not necessarily require combat skills but rather an education-orientated approach.

Law enforcement officers must be able, during their patrols, to educate civilians about the benefits of adhering to the lockdown regulations. The use of force by Namibian police is regulated by the Police Act 19 of 1990, and the provisions of section 14(10) of this legislation permit the reasonable use of force in crime prevention or effecting a lawful arrest. Furthermore, provisions of Article 49 the Criminal Procedure 51 of 1977 permit the use of reasonable force in order to effect an arrest. The cross-cutting theme in these two Namibian legislative pieces, insofar as the use of force is concerned, is that the force used must be reasonable. In other words, the principle of proportionality must be satisfied where force is used. The benefits of the use of force and consequences that might follow must be at an equilibrium (Hubbard, Van Dijcke, Touré, Cooper & Engelbrecht, 2019). The principle of proportionality was also dealt with by the judiciary in the case of *Matlou v Makhubedu 1978 (1) SA 946 (A)*, where the Appellate Division held that "there must be proportionality between the degree of force used and the seriousness of the crime which the victim is suspected."

In Namibia and South Africa, respectively, the measures put in place to curb the spread of COVID-19 include criminal sanctions. In Namibia, a state of disaster remains in force until it is revoked by the President, while in South Africa, the lack of such legislative oversight resulted in a collective responsibility by cabinet, thus the formation of a National Command Council (Gonese, Shivamba, & Meerkotter, 2020). In the declaration of a state of disaster, the primary concern should be the protection of lives. Article 4 of the Basic Principles on the Use of Force and Firearms by Law Enforcement Officials providesthat police officers shall "as far as possible, apply non-violent means before resorting to the use of force and firearms." On the other hand, Article 7 of this international instrument emphasizes the principle of proportionality in the use of force. It is the fundamental duty of governments to ensure implementation of the laws in line with international standards so as to refrain from subjecting people to inhumane and degrading punishment. Furthermore, cases of police brutality must be investigated and prosecuted. The existence of great legislative pieces is meaningless if their implementation is not carried out in light of respect for and promotion of human rights. The issue in South Africa and Namibia is not per se the laws but the socioeconomic fabric stained by corruption, which galvanizes the lack of accountability for law enforcement officers who violate human rights.

On April 4, 2022, the Office of the Presidency in South Africa published a statement in which it announced the termination of the lockdown. According to the statement, South Africa endured 750 days of lockdown, which were implemented at various levels. These vary from levels 1 to 5, guided by, amongst other things, the increase or decrease in numbers of COVID-19 cases and the World Health Organization. About a month prior to the announcement of the termination of the national lockdown, the Socio-Economic Rights Institute (SERI) made a call for the implementation of the Panel of Experts Report on Policing and Crowd (Commission of Inquiry into the Marikana Massacre) (Mabuza, 2022). The call was pursuant to the murder of one Mtokozisi Ntumba, who was fatally shot with a rubber bullet during a students' protest on March 10, 2021 (Simelani, 2022). The deceased was not even part of the protest; he was in fact at a doctor's appointment when he was shot and killed by law enforcement officers during crowd management (Mabuza, 2022). The death of Mthokozisi drew attention and had tongues waging over the use of force and the trigger-happy nature of law enforcement officers. Four police officers were arrested and charged with the murder of Mthokozisi, and the accused police officers were later acquitted (Patrick, 2022). The charges were dropped because the police officers accused of the deceased's murder could not be positively identified in the footage provided to the court (Patrick, 2022). This is yet another classical case highlighting the level of impunity of police brutality and the inappropriate use of force.

CONCLUSION

Civilians do not have power when compared to the police, hence the latter is mandated to protect the former (Lawson, 2013, 219). In cases where there are misconducts on the part of the police, consequences shall follow because, without uncountability, we cannot speak about democratic policing (Kollapen, 1993, 6). Police brutality and use of excessive force do not only violate humans; they also erode the justice system and cause issues of trust between the community and police. What happened to Mr. Khosa would not have happened if the police, including those involved in the Marikana Massacre, were held accountable for the murder of 34 mine workers. The pattern of stories of police brutality in South Africa expounds daily, and there are seldom any recursions against the police involved (Kollapen, 1993, 5). Furthermore, one cannot completely avoid the apartheid racial set-up existing parallel to constitutionalism, where it is the poor black majority of the country who fall victim to police brutality. Apart from adhering the to the Constitution and other relevant laws, law enforcement agencies must change the manner in which they police townships and rural areas in this country (Vincent & Rinella, 1968, 773). South African soldiers and police need a more human rights-based approach when enforcing the laws, including the lockdown regulations. It is worrisome that just three days into the lockdown, the IPID confirmed that it is investigating three deaths that allegedly occurred at the hands of the police (Karrim, 2020). Furthermore, the United Nations Human Rights Office warned against the "heavy-handedness and militarized approach" when enforcing the lockdown laws (Karrim, 2020).

In summation, the enforcement of laws must be guided by the Constitution, relevant international human rights treaties, and domestic laws. Where there is failure by the soldiers and police to adhere to the relevant laws when performing their official duties, accountability must be seen to materialize. The state and its representatives (police and soldiers) are not above the law. While the COVID-19 took the African continent and across globe by storm, human rights violations through police and military brutality did not stop the spread of the virus. In the first few days of the lockdown, more people died in the hands of police as opposed to dying as a result of the novel coronavirus (Karrim, 2020). After 26 years in democracy, the South African police appear to not have been trained and conscientized about human rights and enforcing laws within the confines of the Constitution. Similarly, after 30 years of independence, the Namibian law enforcement officers seem to have no regard for human rights or guiding laws and principles on the use of force. Moreover, our soldiers' behavior and approach to enforcing the lockdown rules are blood-chilling because our soldiers are deployed in several other countries on the African continent as peacemakers. We cannot continue to "hang our heads in shame" due the heavy-handedness and militarized behavior of law enforcement agencies, which violate the very human rights of the people they ought to protect. Cruel, degrading, and inhumane punishment and police brutality are exacerbated by the state's failure to promptly and impartially investigate and prosecute those responsible for such acts. Dissel and Tait (2011, 1) argue that "police that uphold a human rights culture and enforce the law consistently, contribute towards faith in a democracy."

REFERENCES

African Charter on Human and Peoples' Rights 1987.

African Policing Civilian Oversight Forum, Policing Human Rights; Assessing South African.

Brogden, M. Reforming Police Powers in South Africa. *Police Studies: The International Review of Police Development*, 17(1), (1994), 25–44.

Constitution of the Republic South Africa, 1996.

Constitution of the Republic of Namibia, 1990.

Countries' Compliance with the SARPCCO Code of Conduct for Police Officials (2012).

Covid-19 Anti-Repression Working Group. (2020). SA Needs to Restrain Use of Force by Police. Retrieved from https://mg.co.za/author/c19-peoples-coalition-anti-repression-working-group/. (Accessed on 6 September 2022).

Criminal Procedure Act 51 of 1977, Republic of South Africa.

Criminal Procedure Act 51 of 1977, Republic of Namibia.

Defense Act 42 of 2002.

Disaster Management Act 57 of 2002.

Dissel, A. & Tait, S. Implementing the Southern African Regional Police Chiefs Cooperation Organisation. African Policing Civilian Oversight Forum (2011).

F v Minister of Safety and Security 2012 (1) SA 536 CC.

Fact Check Namibia. Police Brutality in Namibia. (2020). Retrieved from https://namibiafactcheck.org.na/reports/. (Accessed on 12 August 2020).

Faull, A. At a Time When National Unity and the Cooperation of All Citizens is Vital, Such Actions Could Prove Disastrous. (2020). Retrieved from https://issafrica.org/crimehub/iss-today/state-abuses-could-match-the-threat-of-covid-19-itself. (Accessed on 6 September 2020).

Foster, D. & Luyt, C. The Blue Man's Burden: Policing the Police in South Africa. *South African Journal on Human Rights*, 2(3), (1986), 297–311.

Gawanas, S. S. The LPM Aims to Restore the Dignity of the Namibian People through Mobilization of the Masses to Stand Up for Their Rights and Root Out Corruption. (2020). Retrieved from https://progressive.international/wire/2020-06-01-the-landless-peoples-movement-namibia-in-lockdown/en. (Accessed on 2 September 2022).

Good Governance Africa, Patrolling during a Pandemic, Recommendations to the South African Police Service and South African National Defence Force during the COVID-19 Deployment (May 2020).

Gonese, T., Shivamba, A. & Meerkotter, A. South African Litigation Centre, SALC Brief Policy 1 2020. Legal Overview of COVID-19 on Justice and Right in South Africa (2020).

Gumede, W. Complaints against SANDF. (2020). Retrieved from https://www.wits.ac.za/covid19/covid19-news/latest/complaints-against-sandf.html. (Accessed on 6 September 2020).

Haysom, N. Licence to Kill Part I: The South African Police and the Use of Deadly Force. *South African Journal on Human Rights*, 3(1), (1987), 3–27.

Head, T. Watch: Free State Mayor Tells SANDF to 'Skop' Citizens in Offensive Rant. (2020). Retrieved from https://www.thesouthafrican.com/news/offbeat/watch-matjhabeng-mayor-sandf-speech-skop-donder-video/. (Accessed on 6 September 2020).

Heywood, M. Human Rights, the Rule of Law, and COVID-19 in South Africa. (2020). Retrieved from https://blog.petrieflom.law.harvard.edu/2020/06/04/south-africa-global-responses-covid19/. (Accessed on 24 August 2023).

Hubbard, D., Van Dijcke, H., Touré, Cooper, A. & Engelbrecht, Y.; Legal Assistance Centre. Use of Force by Law Enforcement Officials in Namibia (2019).

Independent Police Investigative Directorate, Annual Report 2012/13 (2013).

International Covenant on Civil and Political Right 1966.

Izobo, M. & Abiodun, F. Enforcement of Lockdown Regulations and Law Enforcement Brutality in Nigeria and South Africa. (2020). Retrieved from https://www.dailymaverick.co.za/article/2020-05-08-lockdown-violence-by-law-enforcement-officials-is-a-throwback-to-a-brutal-past/. (Accessed on 24 March 2021).

Karrim, A. Covid-19: UN Human Rights Office Concerned by Excessive Force, Death Reports during SA Lockdown. (2020). Retrieved from https://www.news24.com/news24/southafrica/news/un-human-rights-office-highlights-toxic-lockdown-culture-in-sa-20200428. (Accessed on 26 March 2021).

Khosa Mpepu & Others v Minister of Defence and Military Veteran & Others 21512/2020.

Kings, S. Why Cops Accused of Killing Tatane Walked Free. (2013). Retrieved from https://mg.co.za/article/2013-03-28-tatane-cops-acquitted-after-messy-case/. (Accessed on 6 September 2020).

Knoetze, D. IPID's Cover-up of Police Brutality in SA. (2019). Retrieved https://www.news24.com/news24/southafrica/news/ipids-cover-up-of-police-brutality-in-sa-20191008. (Accessed on 6 September 2020).

Kollapen, N. N. Accountability: The Debate in South Africa. *Journal of African Law*, 37(1), (1993), 1–9.

Lawson, T. F. Powerless against Police Brutality: Felon's Story. *St. Thomas Law Review*, 25(2), (2013), 218–243.

Mabuza, E. Mthokozisi Ntumba's Death by Rubber Bullet was Avoidable. https://www.timeslive.co.za/news/south-africa/2022-03-10-mthokozisi-ntumbas-death-by-rubber-bullet-was-avoidable-rights-institute/. (Accessed on 8 January 2023).

Matlou v Makhubedu 1978 (1) SA 946 (A).

Mutua, M. Hope and Despair for a New South Africa: Limits of the Rights Discourse. *Harvard Human Rights Law Journal*, 10(63), (1997), 1057–5057.

Namibia Fact Check (2020) Spotlight. (Accessed on 12 August 2020).

Optional Protocol to the United Nations Convention Against Torture 2006.

Panel of Experts Report on Policing and Crowd Management Established by the Minister of Police in Terms of the Recommendations of the Marikana Commission of Inquiry (2018).

Patrick, A. Cops Accused of Mthokozisi Ntumba's Death Acquitted. https://www.timeslive.co.za/news/south-africa/2022-07-05-cops-accused-of-mthokozisi-ntumbas-death-acquitted/. (Accessed on 8 January 2022).

Police Act 19 of 1990.

Prevention of Combating and Torture of Persons Act 13 of 2013.

Sidimba, L. Police Minister Bheki Cele Appeals Portion of Collins Khosa Ruling. (2020). Retrieved from https://www.iol.co.za/news/politics/police-minister-bheki-cele-appeals-portion-of-collins-khosa-ruling-48999920. (Accessed on 21 July 2021).

South African History Online. The Namibian Struggle for Independence – 1966–1990 – a Historical Background. (2020). Retrieved from https://www.sahistory.org.za/article/namibian-struggle-independence-1966-1990-historical-background. (Accessed on 6 September 2020).

South African Police Services Act 68 OF 1995.

Southern African Regional Police Chiefs Cooperation Organisation Code of Conduct of the Police Officials 1995.

Statement by President Cyril Ramaphosa on the Termination of the National State of Disaster in Response to the Covid-19 Pandemic. (Accessed on 8 January 2023).

Treatment of Punishment 1984.

United Nations Basic Principles on the Use of Force and Firearms by Law Enforcement Officials 1990. Universal Declaration of Human Rights 1948.

United Nations Convention Against Torture and Other Cruel, Inhumane and Degrading.

Use of Force and Torture: Guideline on the Implementation and Enforcement of Regulations and Directives Issued in Terms of Section 27 of the Disaster Management Act, 2002 (Act no. 57 of 2002): Containment and Management of COVID-19.

Vincent, J. & Rinella, V. J. Police Brutality and Racial Prejudice: First Close Look. *Journal of Urban Law*, 45(Issues & 4), (1968), 773–804.

Wekili, S. & Leus, H. E. Police Brutality: Problems of Excessive Power Litigation. *Pacific Law Journal,* 25(2), (1994), 171–210.

Chapter 4

Civil-Military Relations and Internal Security

Question of Ethics and Security

Mabuku Kaumba Kennedy and
Masake Pilisano Harris

INTRODUCTION

The central focus of the chapter is on military participation in COVID-19-led operations and internal security. Governments around the world deployed their military forces to respond to the COVID-19 pandemic. The premise of this approach emphasizes that the suppression of internal disasters is not exclusive but rather a concerted effort. This chapter argues that the military's involvement in internal police pandemic-led operations has negative and positive implications for the citizens. It further argues that the benefits associated with military involvement in internal operations outweigh the insecurities caused by its involvement. Furthermore, this chapter predicts the emergence of a new security era referred to as the Fused Security Era.

The growing utilization of the military in any part of the world is often attributed to the widening gap between the needs of affected populations, resource demands, and the capacity of civilian actors to fulfil both rapid and large-scale emergencies and disasters (Musa, 2018). In addition to the above, there are several possible explanations for increased military involvement in operations and patrol within the domestic setting. Firstly, health care has become strained and plagued by the overall effects of COVID-19. Secondly, law enforcement agencies struggle with limited personnel in terms of deploying their available personnel between crime prevention and deterrent initiatives, crime investigations, crime detection, and enforcement of pandemic regulations. Lastly, the incessant insecurities practices necessitated by internal factors.

With the pandemic waging war on the existence of humanity, governments had to take a serious stance and intensify their approaches to mitigate its effects. It is common practice that the state's primary responsibility is the protection of its citizens against peripheral aggression and internal insecurities. The latter is the mandate of the police in liberal democracies, for instance, in Namibia. The second amendment to the Namibian Constitution provides, under Article 118, the establishment of the Namibian Police with prescribed powers, duties, and procedures to preserve Namibia's internal security and maintain law and order. However, as violence erupts and the security situation deteriorates, regimes often rely on deploying the military to enforce orderliness and the return of peace, as well as the eradication of human security threats in all its dimensions. This is largely because police are unable to ultimately preserve internal security, especially where the citizenry's personal, food, community, and health security are threatened by other factors, both human-motivated and natural trends. The pandemic outbreak, as stated earlier, concedes well with the preceding notion.

As the effects of COVID-19 were increasingly felt around the globe, several regulations and measures were put in place to address its effects, including the deployment of the military alongside the police. However, the implementation of the regulations set during COVID-19 prompted divided opinions regarding the military's role. Political scientists, human rights activists, and analysts questioned the military's role as part of the response. While there are mixed sentiments on military involvement in the fight against an invisible enemy (COVID-19), it is pertinent to note that military units over the years have provided services such as disaster relief in terms of health, education, and other humanitarian efforts when internal service capabilities are insufficient.

However, when armed forces' involvement in domestic affairs occurs, the questions of authorities, military brutality, and the use of firearms become security-related issues. It is clear that the more the military is involved in internal security, the more the likelihood of increased security forces' brutality toward the citizens. This encourages critical thinking about military action and the possible remedies. On this basis, this chapter anticipates the eruption of a new security era where the military's involvement in domestic security will be understood and not questioned by ordinary citizens. The prediction of the new security era is pinned on the principle that insecurities within and outside the territorial borders of the states will only effectively be addressed with bonded efforts from security forces, that is, the military, police, and other stakeholders. This is certainly true, given the already visible police-military-led operations and patrols in various countries even before the outbreak.

THEORY ON MILITARY INVOLVEMENT IN DOMESTIC AFFAIRS

In the pursuit to extend our understanding of the involvement of the military in COVID-19 operations and internal security in general, it is prudent to discuss theories that govern military involvement in internal security. Furthermore, the theory is compelled by the need to successfully surmount any obstacles limiting comprehension of the question of integrating the military into the police officer's role. Therefore, even though several theories are used for military involvement in internal security, integration theory may be appropriate for this chapter.

Morris Janowitz, a military sociologist, developed the integration theory that focused on the professional stature of the military and its changing role in a globalized society. He contended that the military profession prescribes a well-defined structure, rules, and self-induced professional standards, ethics, and norms (Janowitz, 1960, p. 420). This ensures that the military remains obedient to the rule of law, and he asserts that civilian control of the military can only be achieved when the military is integrated into society and the political decision-making processes. There are several possible explanations for this theory's importance to military involvement in COVID-19 police-led operations and internal security. One of them is that it may assist military personnel themselves to be more passionate and empathetic with civilian components and hone their ability to forge interpersonal relationships during their involvement in internal security. Subsequently, they ensure that they strive to treat public members with the utmost respect, taking into account not straying from human rights violations.

Besides, the integration theory advocate for a mental twist; for military personnel to understand civil society operations, structural change needs to be realized. This argument is supported by CashMan (2018), who warns that if there is no transformation inside each of us, then structural change in the world would be an impossible mandate. However, it must be noted that operation and structural change are only possible if the act of integration is at the epitome of any entity. One of these is the changing pattern of security problems, which has meant that the military is used increasingly in constabulary roles. Implying that the military is used in an internal role in several states, blurring the lines between policing and military functions and between peace and war. Namibia provides a typical example of the role of military involvement in internal security. With increased crime rates, accelerated insecurities, and gang activities in the country, in 2018, Operation "Hornkranz" was launched, which was followed by Kalahari and Namib Desert operations launched in 2019.

These operations combine members of the army and police force as well as other stakeholders working together in patrolling the street, arresting the offenders, and maintaining law and order in general. Since then, there have been several joint police-led operations. The present simultaneous operation started in 2021 is "Operation Hokanam," and all these operations are presumed to leapfrog the COVID-19 era (Nangolo, 2020). These sorts of interactions are further strengthened by military personnel's involvement in the COVID-19 police-led operations. The preceding arguments hold relevance as it has been seen over the centuries that military involvement in internal security has become a more prominent and undeniable endeavor. With the pandemic outbreak, it is no surprise that we have seen even more military involvement in internal security than ever before. Given this, it is imperative that the military, during their operations within states, share, respect, and embrace the democratic values that society enjoys (Harig, Jenne, & Ruffa, 2022). Where the military shares the democratic values of society, it will be more committed to achieving the political goals of the state (Janowitz, 1977, p. 73).

MILITARY ROLE IN COVID-19-LED OPERATIONS AND INTERNAL SECURITY

There are some counterarguments to the deployment of defense forces in domestic affairs. To begin with, the military has been trained and equipped for precisely the opposite of saving lives (Yılmaz & Ağkaya, 2022). Its purpose is to defend the country and its people against physical and external enemies by subduing such enemies if need be. Despite these mandatory functions, the role of the military has been expanded. Already, today, reports around the globe clearly show that armed forces are providing unmatched assistance within their states in the struggle to curtail the world pandemic of the novel coronavirus and preserve internal security, as mentioned already. It is now well established that the national armies have been equipped to set up more hospital capacity and provide their mobile clinics. Also, using the expertise within the military to serve lives and assume the role of medics, transporting supplies, and providing other logistics needs, as well as patrolling the streets to enforce the regulations.

The preceding is particularly true given the limited number of police personnel in general. The above means that the police population ratio compared to the Namibian population is estimated to be one police official per 164 citizens. To illustrate the police understaffed security concern, Kenya and Ghana provide relevant examples. The United Nations recommends one police officer for every 450 citizens (Amuya & Mwai, 2016). In Kenya, a police official serves 1,150 citizens (Amuya & Mwai, 2016). While in Ghana, the ratio of police official to citizen is estimated to be one police official for every 1,161 citizens (Appiahene-Gyamfi, 2021). The preceding bears implications as understaffed police organizations may partly explain their inability to preserve internal security effectively caused by any factors or COVID-19, hence the need for stakeholders' involvement, such as the military.

The spread of COVID-19 requires the wide spread of law enforcement officers and armies to present a solution to the already existing crisis of human resources. Besides, the presence of armies in the streets serves as a deterrent to compliance with the regulations set for addressing the pandemic. It is believed by the public members that military uniform and equipment with all the accessories institute fears among the population. This notion is particularly true given the number of brutalities and atrocities committed by military members as a result of patrolling the streets. In view of all that has been mentioned so far, one may suppose to ask one pertinent question: are the threats caused by military presence on the street patrols during the pandemic outweighing the role that they play in combating the pandemic? In answering this question, we may again remind ourselves about the military's role during the pandemic.

Firstly, operating in a supplementary role, armed forces' participation in internal security tasks aims at mitigating the shortfall of local police forces' manpower, relieving them of more demanding tasks. For example, in Spain, the army has a particular unit (Unidad Militar de Emergencias) that works under the framework of civil protection. In that capacity, its soldiers act under the same legal umbrella as the civilian police, even during peacetime (Yılmaz & Ağkaya, 2022). Furthermore, in African countries, including Namibia, the military has been utilized for street patrols to preserve internal security and the operation of COVID-19. For instance, in an article titled "How far will the government go on using the Namibian military to blackmail civilians before realizing it has gone too far?" published in the Namibian newspaper, it is claimed that over the past three years, "the military presence in towns and villages has grown apace in Namibia due to the insecurities, where Namibian Defense Force assumed a prevalent proactive role in internal safety and security" (*The Namibian*, 2020, p. 11).

These insecurities may explain the relative reason why military patrol streets in quarantine areas persuade citizens to stay at home and enforce social distance compliance. Also, there have been some instances where the military has been deployed in many countries to enforce lockdowns and traffic regulations. When traffic regulations become the center of focus, there can be no doubt that any state's ability to contain the pandemic cannot be realized without regulating traffic movements. Thus, during COVID-19, the restriction of movement from one place to another became a common permissible practice. The reason attributed to this is the willingness of the government to reduce physical contact as much as possible to limit the spread of local transmission of COVID-19.

Nonetheless, the presence of armed forces somewhat increased the level of compliance by the citizens. This is evident given the complaints of public members using all the available communication media to plead with the government to withdraw the military on the street for their free movement. With the above as a backdrop, it is notable that the armies played a significant role in supporting various government efforts of preserving lives, reducing human atrocities, and assisting in the slow spread of infection during the pandemic. As reported by Rozenblum, Greer, Wismar, and Jarman (2020), the military helped in various ways. It focused mostly on ensuring sufficient physical infrastructure by providing medical equipment such as ventilators and ICU beds and ensuring sufficient workforce capacity by sending military physicians to civil hospitals and isolation and quarantine facilities.

INSECURITIES ASSOCIATES AND MILITARY INVOLVEMENT IN DOMESTIC SECURITY

The writers of this chapter felt it pertinent to also discuss the factors linked to insecurities in general and insecurity amidst military presence in domestic security affairs. Carr (1940) argues that the lack of security in the world is caused by differing endowments of resources and governmental structures, conflicting ideologies, and the thirst for power of certain leaders. The opinion seems to be relevant even in today's twenty-first century. For instance, in Middle Eastern countries such as Egypt, Turkey, Saudi Arabia, Morocco, Jordan, Israel, Iraq, Iran, and Algeria, religious differences have often been cited as one of the primary causes of conflicts leading to heightened insecurities among these states (Tamon, 2023). This could be mainly attributed to three main religions: Christianity, Islam, and Judaism. As a result, the Middle East is among the most diverse regions in terms of religions. This variety of beliefs can lead to a difference in opinion and conflicting ideologies, which often leads to religious disputes in the region.

These ideas resounded those of the philosopher Jean-Jacques Rousseau (cited by Walt, 2010, p. 321), who singled out two main factors of insecurity between states: interdependence and inequality. As states become dependent on one another, this creates suspicion and incompatibility, and the unequal allocation of resources helps drive conflict. This has been the case in many African countries where initial observation suggests that, most notably, causes of insecurities result from unequal economic growth that still widens the gap between the rich and poor. Another source of uncertainty is the failure of the government to address challenges that affect the survival of its citizens. This has seen the reoccurrence of insecurities in some countries. Weak governance is observed as another cause of insecurities.

A note of caution is due here since weak governance is often coupled with a weak state, making it challenging to administer sufficient state funds and resources. The claim of weak government as a source of insecurity is supported by (Buzan, 1983, p. 25), who vividly argues that, apart from other sources, the threats of insecurity emerge from sources that are the state itself through its military institutions and poor administration of government affairs or armed groups. In terms of the former, studies show that where the state does not regulate its institutions effectively, they can become a source of insecurity for the citizenry. Such threats include "physical threats (pain, injury, death), economic threats (seizure or destruction of property, denial of access to work or resources), threats to rights (imprisonment, denial of normal civil activities), and threats to position or status (demotion, public humiliation) (Howe, 2001, p. 13). This is true in the case of Mozambique, particularly in Cabo Delgado Province (Mlambo & Masuku, 2022). In addition, the endless selfish desire for power of some individual leaders, prompting them to want to remain in power for so long, is another concern for insecurity.

For Waltz (1981), he does not disagree with the desire for power as associated with insecurity, but he instead adds that states only concern themselves with the pursuit of power after national security has been achieved. Particularly when it comes to ownership of physical goods such as land and property. Taken together, the sentiments noted by Waltz (1981) may mean that, given the factors attributed to insecurities, the existence of the state and its government is not enough without fair access to land and properties by citizens of the country. The latter may worsen during the era of COVID-19 as citizens and countries around the globe adjust to the new normal. Because the government is concentrating on curbing the escalation of the pandemic, issues that have to do with land allocation may not be the state's priority.

The above cannot be contested given the fact that food can only be produced through the availability of land; an improved economy is most likely linked to the land. It is crucial to keep in mind that, through agricultural land, more production of goods and services is realized, which contributes to the GDP of any given country.

The various factors of insecurities have created grievances and opportunities for violence that have changed the nature of security threats in the world. The discussion above provides the answers as to why the military is seen in some instances to address challenges of insecurities. It is arguable not that the armies' training emphasizes killing the enemies, and their mindset becomes predominantly preoccupied by brutality in all their undertakings. Given our combined police experience of 34 years, this assertion could be true that the armies are well trained to counter the adversaries. It is evident that the types of training a person undergo determine how a person reacts to situations. It is within these realms that military involvement in domestic security presents insecurity to the populace. Insecurities surrounding the military in domestic security could be segmented into two groups. First, those associated with overall military performance and the effects on the population's interaction.

It is almost certain that in the twenty-first century, military's role is expanded to, among others, putting more emphasis on peacekeeping missions necessitated by a reality check that positions security practitioners and political elite to understand that peace, to a large extent, can be achieved through peaceful means. The latter practice is attributed to the persistence of deployed armed forces abroad in peacekeeping missions and conflict resolution missions. Due to the pandemic outbreak, initial evidence also suggests that military deployment is temporarily scaled down while in some countries it has been stooped completely, affecting their role in preserving peace in the international arena.

The outbreak of the pandemic attracted more military involvement to provide support to the government in domestic security, which was previously known as the police responsibility only, while at the same time reducing military role abroad. The other common reasons cited for the reduced number of deployments of armies abroad are fear of contracting the virus, closed borders, diverting resources to compress the pandemic, and the need for increased local deployment of the military. Some analysts and scholars may applaud the move to scale down the military forces abroad as a means to save funds and resources. It is, however, important to highlight that this may exacerbate insecurities experienced in some countries. Because the global sphere is interdependent, conflicts or uncertainty in other parts of the globe directly or indirectly affect the socio-economic interaction of other peaceful nations. Consequently, it threatens the existence of humanity.

The advancement of military forces in domestic security affairs has to be carefully considered. Bergman, Mackay, and Pell (2021) posit that the requirement to provide operational support to the civilian government during large-scale civil emergencies is the source of insecurities for professional militaries. Especially if this undermines their ability to perform priority functions in external defense. Tasking the armed forces as an auxiliary emergency service incurs some opportunity cost in terms of defense readiness and maintaining skills for warfighting. This is so because one visible implication and insecurity is the context within which the political elite have encroached in the military domain to dictate how the military should operate, posing the greatest threat to national security. Due to the significant impact of the COVID-19 pandemic, it is likely that military commanders are placing increased emphasis on the aspect of safeguarding their workforces deployed in COVID-19 frontline operations.

As previously elucidated in this chapter, it becomes clear that insecurities related to the military's role in the COVID-19 operation are visualized by observing them within the military organogram. While lessening the impact of COVID-19 on human security has been the priority of governments around the globe, the act has never been easier for military forces.

There are forms of resistance and compliance with the state of emergence by some portion of the public members. The implications of this resistance have seen an increase in security forces using emergency powers as a weapon to quash dissent and control the population. In this context, such actions often involve significant violations of human rights, resulting in inflicting of pain and in some instance causing death. As reported recently by BBC News, for instance, in Nigeria, in first two months, security forces enforcing the lockdown in parts of Nigeria killed more people than the number of people that died from coronavirus. Also, Nigeria has been prevalently deploying the military to deal with issues related to internal security and law enforcement operations since the independence of the country in 1960 (Joshua, Gberevbie, & Onor, 2021). Due to its ever-omnipresence in internal affairs, it has become a significant player in politics, as Nigeria has been under military rule for about 29 years (Ediagbonya, 2019). It could be right to mention that the situation surrounding military involvement in internal security may exacerbate the already-existing insecurities faced in several countries.

Guided by the preceding thoughts, the relevance of integration theory becomes more and more clear. The idea of involving military personnel in domestic security to address challenges to public peace and citizen satisfaction was embraced by politicians, political scientists, scholars, and youth activists. However, this notion has been met with practical controversy, and Nigeria's situation serves as partial evidence to the contrary. The initial observation is that prolonged military participation in internal security affairs does not guarantee the internalizing of social values that support citizen sovereignty and uphold and respect the rule of law as well as democratic culture. It could be stated that the integration process of the military into civil duties lacks implementation. Hence, the reason for the failure of armies to adapt to civil duties while taking cognizance of their obligations. Incorporating the military into the COVID-19 police-led operations should be a thoughtful endeavor that requires support. The lack of proper methods and planning for integrating military personnel into domestic civil affairs and addressing anticipated concerns within the state will be a far-fetched reality. With the above, questions may emerge: could the failure to integrate military personnel through integration theory be one reason why some public members still despise using military participation in internal security? The above narratives provide us with something to ponder.

The pandemic has meant that the security cluster, including the military, works under more constant stress than before while attempting to enforce adherence to regulations and guidelines as pronounced in each country. Thus, constant confrontation with such social problems puts some members of the military, who are only trained to attack enemies, under psychological strain, leading them to resort to brutality that results in injuries, psychological trauma, or death to the general public (Tejada & Gorling, 2017). These acts are contrary to the security cluster's anticipated most crucial job of preserving human life while maintaining order. Given the unfriendly experiences that the citizenry endures when interacting with the military, most of the populace fears encountering soldiers (Mabuku, 2023). Adding to this, the citizenry experiences fear because military abuse is a continuous threat in their everyday lives. Just as it has been the case in the implementation of lockdown regulations, military personnel brutalize the public, instituting further insecurities. This accounts for the several impediments and discrepancies experienced when the military is involved in an internal role. To this end, a noble and respected security force task that comes with great accountability and responsibility has been tested to the core during COVID-19.

MILITARY ROLE IN INTERNAL SECURITY OPERATION A NEW NORMAL

Over the years, there has been an observable increase in military participation in the domestic-led operations of several countries. The practice is no longer a surprise, given that the view of security and security threats has expanded. For instance, protecting the nation from external aggressors, invaders, threats, or turbulent global economic waves is no longer justifiable without extending security arms to include human security domestically.

Today, it is undeniable that the biggest security threats to the existence of mankind are no longer an external army but domestic threats. This plausible understanding may be a reason why the military role in internal security has extended to encroach the domestic realm. The relevancy of the backdrop could further be grasped within Pion-Berli (2017, p. 103). Arguments, natural disasters, environmental degradation, undocumented immigration, and even extreme poverty are often portrayed as events or processes that could, if left unattended, materialize into security threats, even crises.

The criminal activities are increasingly coordinated, large in scope, and transnational or cross-border in nature. For the reason that these types of insecurities have shifted from being external-centric only to internal-centric, in the end, attracting and capturing military focus on internal security. For example, to maintain that military participation in COVID-19-led operations is unjustifiable is to make a mockery of the human security threat posed by COVID-19. This raises an intriguing question regarding the nature and extent of the question of whether the military is suitable for domestic security affairs. This question could be answered by the background on the military's role in the COVID-19 era and years beyond, as alluded to earlier in this chapter. Even though there is a sharp division that exists among scholars, conditioned by years of training and indoctrination, soldiers seek and destroy an enemy. The notion is still dominant in the twenty-first century that soldiers do not protect and serve a citizenry role.

It may be the case; however, it has become apparent that this belief is slowly losing its stance given the changing nature of human security threats. Therefore, in the foreseeable future, a change in military training to include aspects of human rights, internal interactions, and internal operations will be imminent.

It can be also anticipated that law enforcement agencies will undergo a more extensive form of military-style training, while armed forces will include elements of police training in their preparations, even beyond the pandemic era, with all parties involved as stakeholders.

In general, therefore, it seems that the cohesion and mutual functions of both the armies and police will be integrated into various facets. The possibility of a new era surfacing where the military will be a friendly entity with more concern for the lives of its citizens than merely killing enemies cannot be ruled out. During this era, military operations internally will be a normal endeavor; citizens will accept military involvement in domestic internal operations without questioning their legitimacy. Meanwhile, the armies and the police will form a formidable force congested by the thoughts of the well-being of citizens and national security in general.

The said era will be referred to as the *Fused Security Era.* Founded on the principle that insecurities within and outside the territorial borders can only be addressed with bonded efforts from both security forces, the armies, and the police. Informed by the fused security era, the "flying geese" security pattern will be predominant. The era will be characterized by the integration of four key elements known as Civil-Military Training, Merged Functions, Porous Operational Terrain, and Integrated Security Policy (MPIC), as depicted below:

Civil-Military Training

Civil-military training will involve military training that incorporates, among other civil rights of individuals. Apart from training on counteracting enemies, the training shall emphasize peace operations within the states and civil rights coordination. The training shall shape the military personnel in broadly understanding security, humanitarian, and other areas to attain more extensive, more strategic national security goals. Their mindset comprehends that national security cannot be achieved without the peaceful interaction of citizens in some domestic affairs. This explains the concepts and principles of civil-military training to focus also on human rights and civil interaction within the parameter of national security from a wider, full-spectrum perspective.

Porous Territorial Terrain

The question of porous territorial terrain explores the practical application of the current segmented topographical operation. As human security threats encroach the international domain to breed substantial well within the states, strategic ideas at the operational and tactical levels compel the military to divide their focus. Drawing our attention to the importance of considering porous terrain, the current transnational security threats, such as food, health, community, personnel, and economic and political insecurity, reside within the states. This implies that insecurities threatening human existence before, during, and after pandemic era are within the boundaries of the national border. Apart from the aforementioned threats, weapons of mass destruction, organized crime, terrorism, cybercrime, and natural and human-made disasters are not confined outside the borders and pose, among other greatest threats to national security. These pull factors are among the reasons for military intervention in domestic human security undertakings.

Integrated Security Policy

Integrated Security Policy is designed for military and police personnel to better understand military-police security operation coordination. The legislation provides for the establishment of a framework that incorporates civilian control of the military and demilitarize the police force/service. Both security policies review the importance of work-integrated effort, acknowledging that there is no isolated incidence in terms of security but a combination of different factors that can only be amicably redressed with the consented security policy. It does not drive away totally from the state's security but takes cognizance of a people-centered security approach.

This observation is no longer a surprise for the reason that contemporary global engagements constantly evolve, compelling social interaction to change as well. The insecurities surrounding human existence have crossed borders; human threats are no longer seen in the realm of external aggressors, adversaries, or rivals only, and internal threats have become dominant in recent times.

Merged Functions

The merged functions between the military and the police are the last component. Although there can be no doubt that the military and police will still maintain their principal functions separately, most of the functions are projected to be merged. There are two possible explanations for the projection. In the first place, deterring enemies from entering the territorial border of the state. Initially, the function was previously known to be managed by the military. However, in recent years, the police force has taken the commanding position in establishing bases alongside the borders, patrolling the borders, and becoming the first line of a deterrent. Secondly, the prevalent street patrols and joint security operations of the police and armies to prevent crimes, the preservation of internal security and maintenance of law order, and traffic control duties in many countries serve as a shred of evidence on the possibility of merging the functions of the military and the police. These functions could be incorporated into both police and military policy, as illustrated already, to give effect to the role that both security clusters need to play to curtail human security threats, of which COVID-19 is one of the examples.

POST-COVID-19 IMPLICATIONS

Keeping in par with the new rules of engagement necessitated by COVID-19, the roles of today's armed forces are solely not limited to combat roles anymore; they are now broadened, diverting from concentrating on conventional wars to including crisis response operations within the national boundaries and abroad, which has transcended to post-COVID-19. It is now evident that more people have started appreciating the role that the military plays in internal operations and security in general. Even though a portion of the population still does not favor military involvement in the post-COVID-19-led operation, postmodern military organizations, particularly on operations engagements, have become appealing, carrying out this mandate in close cooperation with police and other security organizations. Initially, armies' involvement in internal operations was seen as a temporary measure many years ago. Meanwhile, the evidence today, even post-COVID-19, suggests that the engagements have become permanent, partly because of the support of some public opinion towards that kind of mission.

As we anticipate more and more waves of change concerning insecurities as the result of human evolution leading to increased security concerns and crises, it may be noble to predict that the military and the police will even closely operate together in the foreseeable future. With this understanding, it was projected that the new era would come to pass in this chapter. The era is referred to by the author as the *Fused Security Era*. In an era in which military operations internally will be a regular endeavor, citizens will accept military involvement in domestic internal operations without questioning their legitimacy.

CONCLUSION

There is no contention that the armies and the police formed formidable forces congested by the thoughts of the well-being of citizens and national security in general during COVID-19. The internal engagement was accepted by the armies, the police, and the public. While there is still a visible sign of resistance from the side of military themselves, police, and some public members, the thinking will soon change as the concept of the Fused Security Era erodes and dominates public opinions. In the final analysis, military involvement in the COVID-19 operation was a sign of relief to others, while others still label its involvement as a threat to national security. Despite positive anticipation that is aligned to the military involvement in COVID-19 in particular and internal security in general, key among the concerns of using the military internally is the lack of preparedness in aligning their operations and rules of engagement. The ability to uphold citizenry liberties on human rights. Even though this is the case, there is no doubt that the benefits of their involvement outweigh the insecurities caused by military involvement in COVID-19. With this in mind, there is a need to support such a move during not only the pandemic but post-pandemic too. Finally, the best way to start is to integrate the military into civil duty by using four components of the Fused Security Era, as illustrated.

REFERENCES

Amuya, L. & Mwai, K. P. Roles of community and police in implementation of community policing: What are the levels of partnership between the community and the police in community policing in Teso South, Busia, Kenya. *International Journal of Novel Research in Humanity and Social Sciences*, 3(6), (2016), 8–19. Retrieved from https://ssrn.com/ abstract=3059230

Appiahene-Gyamfi, J. Policing in Ghana. In Mbuba, J. *Global perspectives in policing and law enforcement: Approaches, challenges and opportunities.* London: Lexington Books (2021), pp. 1–24.

Bergman, B. P., Mackay, D. F., & Pell, J. P. Dementia in Scottish military veterans: Early evidence from a retrospective cohort study. *Psychological Medicine*, (2021), 1–6. http://doi.org/10.1017/S0033291721002440

Branco, C. How armed forces help fight Covid-19. (2020). Retrieved from https://valdaiclub.com/a/highlights/how-armed-forces-help-fight-Covid-19/

Buzan, B. *People, states and fear: The national security problem in international relations*. Brighton: Wheatsheaf Books Ltd (1983).

Carr, E. H. The twenty years crisis, 1919–1939: An introduction to the study of international relations. *University of Chicago Press Journals*, 50(3), (1940), 344–346. Retrieved from https://www.journals.uchicago.edu/doi/10.1086/290162?mobileUi=0

Cashman, K. *Leadership from inside out* (3rd ed.). San Francisco: Berret-Koehler (2018).

Ediagbonya, M. Military administration in Nigeria, 29 years of sad political experience and democratic truncation. *Global Scientific Journal*, 7(8), (2019), 1378–1394.

Harig, C., Jenne, N., & Ruffa, C. Operational experiences, military role conceptions, and their influence on civil-military relations. *European Journal of International Security*, no. 7(1), (2022), 1–17. http://doi.org/10.1017/eis.2021.29

Howe, H. M. *Ambiguous order: Military forces in the African states*. Boulder, CO: Lynne Rienner Publishers (2001).

Janowitz, M. *Military institutions and coercion in the developing nations: The military in the political development of new nations.* Chicago & London: The University of Chicago Press (1977).

Joshua, S., Gberevbie, D., & Onor, K. Building security through insecurity: The Nigerian military and counter-violence campaigns in the fourth republic. *Armed Forces & Society*, 47(1), (2021), 177–200. https://doi.org/10.1177/0095327X209340

Lambert, A. *Democratic civilian control of armed forces in the post-cold war era.* Berlin: LIT Verlag (2009).

Mabuku, K. K. A framework for performing internal security as a constitutional obligation of the namibian police force. PhD Unpublished Thesis (2023). Stadio Higher Education.

Mlambo, V. H. & Masuku, M. M. Terror at the front gate: Insurgency in Mozambique and its implications for the SADC and South Africa. *Journal of Public Affairs* (2022) https://doi.org/10.1002/pa.2700

Musa, Y. S. Military internal security operations in Plateau State, North Central Nigeria: Ameliorating or exacerbating insecurity? [PhD dissertation]. South Africa: Stellenbosch University (2018). https://scholar.sun.ac.za/bitstream/handle/10019.1/1 04931/

Nangolo, F. J. Contribution of the joint operations on crime prevention in Namibia – a case of Wanaheda police station area of jurisdiction in Khomas region

[Master thesis, University of Rwanda]. (2020). http://dr.ur.ac.rw/bitstream/handle/123456789/1083/ NANGOLO %20Frednard%20J..pdf?sequence=1&isAllowed=y

Pion-Berlin, D. The military and internal security operations in Latin America. *Revista Política y Estrategia*, 27(130) (2017), 101–123. https://doi.org/10.26797/rpye.v0i130.131

Rozenblum, S., Greer, S. L., Wismar, M., & Jarman, H. What is the role of the military in the Covid-19 response? (2020). Retrieved from https://analysis.covid-19healthsystem.org/index.php/ 2020/05/29/what-is-the-role-of-the-military-in-Covid-19-response

Tamon, M. L. Conflict analysis in West Asia. *International Journal of Multicultural and Multireligious Understanding*, 10(1), (2023), 230–241.

Waltz, K. The spread of nuclear weapons: More may be better: Introduction. Adelphi Papers 21. (1981). https://doi.org/10.1080/05679328108457394

Yılmaz, A. G. & Ağkaya, O. Military call-out powers and civil-military relations. Military Operation and Engagement in the Domestic Jurisdiction: Comparative Call-out Laws. 2022 June 8:180.

Chapter 5

Security Sector Governance during the State of Emergency and COVID-19 in SADC

Helao Tuhafeni

INTRODUCTION

The extent to which the security sector has been involved in enforcing the laws and state of emergency regulations to assist governments to contain the spreading of the coronavirus (COVID-19) has attracted mixed reactions from the wider community. Domestically, governments have taken drastic measures to safeguard the lives of their citizens against the invisible novel coronavirus (COVID-19). Never before during the post–World War II era, particularly in the Southern African Development Community (SADC), have law enforcement agencies been seized with such catastrophes that made law enforcement officials move closer to the populace and beseech them to abide by the laws. Whereas the security sector has been centrally positioned to assist governments in managing disasters and calamities, policing the COVID-19 pandemic has presented a new philosophical breadth to the security sector in terms of governance, law enforcement, and, inevitably, delivering and promoting safety and security in distraught societies.

The response by the security sectors in the SADC region to enforce the COVID-19-related measures was received with mixed reactions. Security sectors' capacity to deal with the sudden emergence of the pandemic was one aspect in point. While community members have applauded governments' prompt actions and measures to stop the spread of COVID-19 amidst societal strains, they disapproved the actions of some law enforcement agencies. Security sectors' lack of readiness, preparedness, and capabilities to manage the safety and security of people ethically and professionally during the COVID-19 pandemic, especially enforcing the state of emergency regulations, pierced a hollow in law enforcement camouflage. In this regard, security sector governance (SSG) and law enforcement endeavors were exposed in terms of indecisive and inconsistent policing, an unprofessional and unethical approach, and limited capabilities to handle situations of that magnitude, let alone humanely treating persons. The expeditious and swift response by SADC countries in March 2020, that is, Namibia, South Africa, Zambia, and Angola, followed by Botswana in April 2020 to declare a state of emergency, impose lockdowns, and eventually promulgate regulations to guide policing during the pandemic, to a varying degree, left the security sectors with little time to prepare to enter society with confidence and enforce the law and regulations during that testing time. Burger (2020) states that "the rapid steps taken in South Africa to combat the coronavirus didn't allow sufficient planning or training of security forces" (para.1). Basically, the focusing on COVID-19 pandemic calls for inclusive safety and security governance, institutional capacity, proper security sector arrangements and readiness of law enforcement agencies. Therefore, the above accentuates arduous exertions in realizing desired safety and security objectives.

Given the above context, this chapter presents a logical narrative of the nature, scope, and role of the security sector governance in a state of emergency. Moreover, citizens' appreciation of their civic responsibility to support both security sector institutions and the government is indispensable. In this context, the chapter underscores a system thinking approach to the importance and inclusivity of security sector governance. Significantly, the chapter is a narrative on the following: perspective of security sector governance in SADC; security sector preparedness in state of emergency; security sector leadership in the state of emergency; security sector as learning organizations; government approach to safety and security governance; citizens' civic obligation during the state of emergency; and post-COVID-19 implications and way forward.

PERSPECTIVE OF SECURITY SECTOR GOVERNANCE IN SADC

During December 2019, the World Health Organization (WHO) reported a cluster of pneumonia cases in Wuhan City, China. Severe Acute Respiratory Syndrome Coronavirus 2 (SARS-CoV-2) was confirmed as the causative agent of what is known today as COVID-19 (WHO, 2019). This virus or the pandemic has spread around the globe, including the SADC region, at an alarming rate. The outbreak of the pandemic and the attempt to contain it have reinforced and realigned security sector governance around the globe. To put it into context, the concept of security sector governance (SSG) is a buzzword in safety and security administration and management. In the view of Abnother, Fluri, and Jurekovic (2007), the concept alludes to the structures, processes, values, and attitudes that shape decisions about safety and security and their implementation. This is a multilateralized, inclusive, and coordinated approach to the promotion of good governance, effectiveness, and efficiency in the security industry. In the context of this chapter, security sector governance refers to the manner law enforcement activities are organized and governed to support government efforts to mitigate the COVID-19 pandemic and crime in general.

The concept of security governance was adopted in an attempt to build policing institutions that are legitimate, human rights conscious, and operate within the ambit of the constitution and all other guiding laws. Wood (2014) acknowledges several pioneers of policing governance literature, such as Clifford Shearing's concepts of "nodal policing" and "governance of security," which formed "part of the lexicon in a growing body of explanatory and normative work on the development of policing literature across the world" (para.1). Rauch (2000) contends that the adoption of security governance approach introduced a culture of respecting human rights by law enforcement agencies and improved relations between them and the communities they serve. This law enforcement approach underlines what Hoogenwoning (2006) calls "a new shared story" or, as May and Williams (1986) view it "a shared governance" that allows law enforcement leadership and management to refocus and rededicate the organization's attention and efforts toward what works. It also emphasized police obligations as provided in the Police Act, *viz.*, Namibian Police Act of 1990 and the South African Police Service Act of 1995. Policing literature suggests that when security sector governance is properly applied and visionary managed, it can achieve effective security functions, promote the flow of security information, and facilitate speedy decision-making in law enforcement agencies. In this regard, security governance, therefore, appeals for inter-agency coordination and collaboration to contain any disaster or emergency that impedes the nation from living a meaningful life. In other words, security governance presented a rare opportunity for a coordinated approach to policing in an effort to build inclusive outcome-oriented policing. The above understanding seems to fit well with the purpose and intention of policing during public health catastrophes, such as COVID-19. Hylton (2013) advises that policing and law enforcement in a disaster or emergency involve two things: prompt response to the crisis and enforcing the laws or regulations where they are contravened; and providing for the safety and security of the community. These two approaches by Hylton are central to managing crises by law enforcement agencies.

Therefore, in times of disaster or state of emergency like COVID-19, the task of law enforcement ranges from manning fixed roadblocks to regulate and stop the unnecessary movement of people, responding to illegal activities, enforcing the state of emergency regulations, providing support to quarantine facilities, and, in the event of a lockdown, patrolling the streets and rural villages to enforce compliance by affected residents. These are nevertheless not easy tasks and hence require firm and consistent leadership to ensure effective governance of safety and security in society. Equally, policing duties and responsibilities require well-prepared and informed law enforcement officials to handle fragile situations. In a modern democracy, law enforcement is a shared responsibility that can only succeed through a shared vision of inclusive and participatory security governance. In an attempt to put into context the tasks of law enforcement in a democratic setting, Loader (2000) poses a critical question on "how society might best come to terms with . . . and seek to govern . . . the multiplicity of institutional forms that are now involved in the delivery of policing, security services and technologies" (p. 323). As such, contemporary policing and, in fact, effective law enforcement can only prosper if law enforcement agencies adopt and apply democratic policing principles, regardless of what the situation is. In essence, the adoption of a security sector governance approach in the SADC region in the early 1990s has contributed to necessary security reforms that have made it possible for law enforcement to remain relevant to the contemporary situation. In fact, Loader further clarifies that ambiguity by saying that:

> "We are living in the midst of a potentially far-reaching transformation in the means by which order and security are maintained in liberal democratic societies, one that is giving rise to the fragmentation and diversification of policing provision, and ushering in a plethora of agencies and agents, each with particular kinds of responsibility for the delivery of policing and security services and technologies." (p. 323).

Kavari (2020) suggests that law enforcement needs access to the latest policing technology to remain relevant in the fight against crime. This can be done through adopting new ways of fighting crime and continuous development and adaptation. In essence, security governance cuts across all aspects of law enforcement related to administration, management, operations, and other auxiliary services. Law enforcement agencies have a key role to play in both supporting the implementation of public health measures to contain the outbreak and the spreading of the pandemic as well as in preventing specific criminal activities arising from this context (INTERPOL, 2020, p. 8). This is in addition to customary daily policing duties and responsibilities. In other words, the security arrangement on COVID-19-related issues does not negate the traditional police duties. However, Luscombe and McClelland (2020), borrowing from decades of research in criminology, contend that policing interventions related to COVID-19 would not impact all people equally. In this regard, the success of law enforcement strategies is dependent on the government's response to socioeconomic issues in society. Similarly, enforcing the state of emergency or state of national disaster regulations may only succeed if social and economic factors have been addressed.

It is evident that the emergence and spread of COVID-19 in the SADC and worldwide have changed the manner in which law enforcement activities are conducted. It has shifted the police's attention from the traditional way of policing, that is, general crime prevention and investigation, to a more "shared policing": the walk-and-talk, close observation, and, more importantly, pleading with citizens to remain calm, limit their movements, and stay at home. Similarly, COVID-19 has tested law enforcement professionalism, ethics, patience, and capacity to police in an ambiguous situation. Even so, history shows that it has not been easy for law enforcement to conduct their duties without violating human rights. Incidents of harassment, maltreatment of citizens, and excessive use of force have been reported. There have been reports of citizens suffering at the hands of unethical law enforcement officials in South Africa, Namibia, Zimbabwe, as well as other SADC countries. Therefore, effective security sector governance is critical to supporting government efforts to fight COVID-19.

Security sector governance and enforcement of laws during a state of emergency, whether on the streets in urban areas, communities, rural villages, or even manning the country's borders, law enforcement officials are placed at a crossroads in terms of espousing a correct approach to be utilized, if law enforcement agencies are to remain relevant, act professionally, and render effective and efficient policing service. Enforcing the state of emergency and lockdown regulations allows no margin for error. It requires more than just a "law enforcement official." More often than not, police officers, like other persons who provide essential services, are called upon to demonstrate not only professional and quality service but also excellence, fairness, and justice in the process of policing. The following are indispensable, specifically when enforcing the state of emergency or state of national disaster measures:

First, to protect and safeguard the rights of all citizens, irrespective of their social status. In the context of this chapter, the purpose of the state of emergency and lockdown is to protect and save people's lives against the invisible and indiscernible coronavirus and stop the spreading of the pandemic in the SADC region. Whether dealing with economic activities, societal enhancement, or fighting public health crises, human rights should remain inviolable. Security sector institutions are agencies of the state, and as Masake (2019) maintained, the "state bore the [primary] obligation to protect and respect human rights" (p. 150). Ruppel (2009) highlights the importance of protecting and safeguarding human rights in the SADC region to promote regional integration. For him, this is necessary for economic communities in Africa. In the same breath, security governance may be effective in an environment in which human rights are respected and safeguarded. Therefore, carrying out those subtle duties requires law enforcement officials to show a high level of professionalism, more so because they are also putting their lives on the line. In essence, law enforcement during COVID-19 requires proper training, briefing, debriefing, and equipping them with prerequisite knowledge, skills, and competences necessary to perform this essential obligation.

Second, prevent crime and protect citizens' property. The state of emergency brings with it a period of uncertainty. Some businesses and public places were closed, and people were urged to work from home and stay at home, respectively. Essentially, only people who are performing critical (essential) services could be seen here and there. The absence of people at places of business and public spaces presented an opportunity for potential criminals to target those premises as well as other selected places of interest to them. For that reason, law enforcement personnel should at all times maintain a visible presence to deter those with bad intentions from committing crimes. However, this seems not to be the only primary focus of men and women in uniform. There were reports of non-visibility of police officers, especially in rural villages where non-compliance with state emergency regulations has been recorded. The absence of law enforcement in communities and rural villages at this critical time suggests a lack of both capacity and resources to reach all corners of the country. If COVID-19 measures require citizens to be confined at home, there must be an assurance that people's property is safe and intact when they return to work or business. Therefore, law enforcement must redouble efforts and revisit their scope and capacity to effectively prevent crime while at the same time protecting people's property.

Third, disperse gatherings where more than the allowed number of people are in attendance. In response to COVID-19, the World Health Organization (WHO) prescribes "social distancing" as one of the tested measures to prevent the spreading of the pandemic. Enforcing "social distancing" measures requires crowd management skills, good communication skills, interpersonal skills, as well as peacekeeping knowledge. Police action here, though it constitutes law enforcement, should take into consideration the environment, the kind of people found at that place, and the activity being undertaken. It calls for a diplomatic approach to convince the people that what they are doing is not permitted under the state of emergency. In that context, authorities including the police, are called upon to up their game and act ethically and professionally.

Fourth, a professional approach to criminal activities and other incidents emanated from non-compliance with state emergency regulations. Law enforcement officials are believed to have undergone extensive training before being attested as officers. Their actions and behaviors should be beyond reproach. Fundamentally, while the police are regarded as gatekeepers of the criminal justice system (Bittner, 1967; Engel et al., 2017), the manner in which they exercise discretionary powers and selective policing is crucial to the success of government efforts in fighting criminal activities and addressing any volatile situations. Despite the above, the picture some police officers portray in the execution of their duties and responsibilities appears contrary to the letter and spirit of democratic policing. In South Africa, Bruce (2020) equated police action during lockdown to the apartheid-era limitations on the movement of black people in urban areas, saying that even during the 1980 state of emergency, restrictions on people were not so severe. Yes, law enforcement is an essential element of governance. They are needed to contain the situation. Sigsworth (2019) says that "one of the core tenets of democratic policing is that the police help to strengthen the authority of the state" (p. 4). However, as the adage goes, "the police must obey the law while enforcing the law." Therefore, as various policing literature expounds, the action of one indiscipline and recalcitrant police officer may put law enforcement agencies under scrutiny and ultimately tarnish the good image of the police organizations.

Fifth, accountability and transparency in executing police duties and responsibilities. Whether in a state of emergency, lockdown, or other operations, the law enforcement officials are called upon to account for every action they take. Police officers must make ethical decisions. The state of emergency and lockdown do not negate or take away persons' fundamental human rights. Protection of people's lives and liberty, privacy, and dignity must be safeguarded. As indicated earlier, during COVID-19, the primary objective of the state of emergency and state of national disaster was to stop the spreading of the pandemic and manage it to save people's lives. Yes, freedom of movement might be limited; however, that does not necessarily give law enforcement the absolute power to harass, affront, manhandle, and maltreat innocent civilians. Therefore, accountability and transparency are indispensable. In the view of Sigsworth (2019), oversight, accountability, [and transparency] are fundamental elements of democratic policing. In practice, accountability cannot be delegated. Therefore, whatever law enforcement officials do and the manner they behave on the street may reflect on the organization they represent and eventually leadership, hence leadership is accountable for their subordinate misdemeanors. This is not easy at all. The philosophy of "stay out of trouble . . . stifles officers who are otherwise resourceful" (Kelling, 1988, p. 3). To promote accountability, law enforcement leadership should cultivate such an approach through training and development, refresher courses, motivation, proper briefing, and debriefing to develop a formidable police force ready to arrest any undesirable situation. It is within this understanding that security sector governance is at the nerve center of any government during a state of emergency.

SECURITY SECTOR LEADERSHIP PREPAREDNESS IN STATE OF EMERGENCY

The COVID-19 pandemic is the first and worst public health catastrophe to hit the African continent and the SADC region. West Africa (Guinea, Liberia, and Sierra Leone) experienced the outbreak of Ebola virus disease in 2014–2015, which infected 28,000 people and resulted in 11,000 deaths (Graduate Institute Geneva and Global Health Centre, 2015, p. 1). Despite the early warning alert put in place and strengthened after the outbreak of influenza (H1N1) in southern Africa in 2009 (World Health Organization, 2014), COVID-19 has emerged undetected. In this case, however, although some lessons seem to have been learned on how to respond to global public health crises, the preparedness of the security sector in this regard has not been tested before. It should be noted that the state of readiness of the security sector in contributing to the fight against the invisible coronavirus is dependent on alert leadership, resource availability, and the willingness of the government to commit and avail such resources to law enforcement. The capacity of leadership and capabilities of security sector institutions is paramount to handling a state of emergency and disaster. Back in early 2000, Ngoma (2005) cited Peter Vale, who argued that the SADC region lacks an appropriate regional institution[s] to handle security issues. In the same vein, Thompson (in Ngoma, 2005) interrogated the same issue at about the same time and similarly identified that one major dilemma facing (SADC) regional security is the political identity of individuals that is classically understood to lie within the borders of the sovereign state (p. 109). Thompson further argued that while this does not conflict with the state-centric focus of the security community approach, its application to the regional level is seen as problematic. His conclusion, therefore, was that the presumed lack of political identity at the regional level makes the achievement of security at this higher level difficult. Vale and Thompson's arguments cannot be delinked from security sector governance and leadership. For effective and efficient security sector governance to materialize, good security sector governance and leadership are prerequisites. It promotes coordinated security and safety cooperation and collaboration among regional member states, eventually strengthening the security sector's capacity to support government efforts.

The above arguments found relevance in the time of COVID-19, where identical domestic measures are needed. It appears that the shortcomings of the early 2000s continue to haunt SADC. This has been exposed by the outbreak of COVID-19. Regional governments and their respective security sectors failed to contain the spread of COVID-19. Their focus is more on individual communities and people than on putting in place effective law enforcement measures to address the pandemic in the region. COVID-19 cases are on the increase in SADC countries such as South Africa, Namibia, Zambia, and Zimbabwe, despite measures that individual governments have introduced and implemented. It should be noted that following and adhering to the World Health Organization's global measures is one thing, and putting in place and applying an individual country's domestic measures is another. Security institutions such as the defense force, the police, and state security a shoulder demanding, sensitive and obligatory responsibility to defend the country, protect citizens, and make sure that the necessary intelligence has been collected, analyzed, and correctly utilized to make informed decisions. So, security sector leadership's preparedness should not be a matter of doubt. Pro-activeness and prompt response to issues that pose a potential threat to the state and public health should be considered second to none. Unlike general crime and criminal activities, COVID-19 is invisible, and its penetrable approach cannot be detected until the person has tested positive for the coronavirus. Therefore, the prevention and containment of COVID-19 require coordinated regional efforts and security institutions to prepare well in advance. According to Graduate Institute Geneva and Global Health Centre (2015), the involvement of the security sector in public health crises and emergency responses is recurrent and is often seen as a necessity. It is further argued that to succeed in managing national disasters, the security sector should be trusted and respected, and its added value in countering public health crises should be recognized. Therefore, aspects of capacity building, human resources training and development, building an effective security system, building a reliable security safety net, and preparing citizens are some of the indispensable protection measures governments can be employed to be ready for any potential crisis. However, drawing from SADC governments' national budget and expenditure, it is evident that governments spent a fortune on the military rather than balancing the equation. The equation in this context implies capacitating all security sectors, including the national police, local police, security firms, vigilantes, and society at large. This enables the government to promptly respond and succeed in all its efforts. In that context, COVID-19 serves as a practical lesson for future planning and actions. Security sector preparedness cannot be overemphasized in times of emergencies and calamities; therefore, it calls for a learning organization approach.

SECURITY SECTORS AS LEARNING ORGANIZATIONS

The outbreak of COVID-19 and the immense challenge faced by security sector necessitate law enforcement agencies to adopt a "learning organizational approach." The concept of "a learning organization" is in most cases confused with the term "organizational learning" though they may be used interchangeably. Peter Senge, in his various studies on the two concepts, provided a clear distinction between the two (Bratianu, 2015). The explanation that fits well with the context of this chapter is that a learning organization is essentially an organization that is continually expanding its capacity to create its future. Senge argued that it is not sufficient for an organization to merely survive or adapt to the environment. But for a learning organization, "adaptive learning" must be joined by "generative learning," learning that enhances the capacity to create…" design and employ those changes that improve the quality of services and adapt the level of knowledge and performance of an organization to the level of the external environment. According to Senge, all learning is directed towards some desired result, involves the encouragement of thinking and group learning, and is a transformative process (Bratianu, 2015, ch 12, para.1).

The universality of law enforcement practice around the globe suggests that security sectors need to learn from each other and adopt law enforcement approaches that are beneficial to the entire citizenry. A learning security sector builds skills and competences, transforms its duties, and aligns them with contemporary challenges and trends. This underscores the significance of a learning organizational approach in mitigating public health crises like the COVID-19 pandemic.

Formal law enforcement has been in existence since time immemorial. Over the years, uncountable efforts have been made to reform the activities of security sector and strengthen them to effectively respond to global crises. Although there have been some major outbreaks of diseases elsewhere in the world, such as the 1918 Spanish flu, 1956 Asian flu, 2009 Influenza (H1N1), and the Ebola virus in 2014, governments in the SADC region have never before experienced a deadly pandemic like what COVID-19 has presented. In mid-September 2020, six countries in the SADC region (South Africa, Zambia, Zimbabwe, Angola, Namibia, and Botswana) recorded a combined total of 16,007 COVID-19-related deaths (Worldometers, 2020). South Africa recorded the highest (15,265) while Botswana recorded the lowest 10 COVID-19. This disastrous situation has caught both governments and their security sectors unaware and unprepared. For that reason, they had to "pull out all the stops" to mitigate the COVID-19 pandemic. In the context of the security sectors in the SADC region, dealing with public health issues is a new concept; hence, for policing institutions it has been a trial-and-error approach.

But the central questions here are: what have security sector agencies learned from the 1918 Spanish flu, 1956 Asian flu, 2009 Influenza H1N1, and 2014 Ebola, and their devastating effects? What lessons would security sector learn from COVID-19 experience? How would the pandemic prepare security institutions to deal with future disasters? Or, as Dag Hammarskjold

Foundation (2012) illustrated on the notion of "the rise of global disaster management," what is the right way to address emergencies and disasters? Although the above-mentioned public health crises have not taken place in the SADC region, policing is universal, and as learning institutions, law enforcement agencies are expected to learn from each other in an effort to prepare for future eventualities. Security sectors in the SADC region could have learned from the above situation.

Institutionalizing security sector governance would be an effective approach to addressing the above questions. Similarly, adopting "what works" (WHO, 2014) could place security institutions in an advantageous and strategic position and prepare them to respond to emergencies and disasters. In this regard, security governance should take on board the people, other stakeholders, and entire citizenship to contain public health crises. In a time of crisis, "people matter" (Helao, 2015). Yes, other resources are equally important, but it is the people who should make a difference in risk and disaster management. Therefore, as it is argued in this chapter, COVID-19 has presented a unique opportunity for security sectors to adopt a learning organizational approach that gives them a unique opportunity to learn while practicing safety and security duties and responsibilities, creating capacity, building a security community, coordinating efforts, and assuming a firm but strategic position to support government efforts and be resolute in addressing issues that affect both human rights and public health issues. Garvin, Edmondson, and Gino, cited in Bratianu (2015), suggested an assessment tool for learning organizations to measure their degree of learning. These are: a supportive learning environment; concrete learning processes and practices; and leadership that reinforces learning.

Considering and adopting Gavin, Edmondson, and Gino's approach could help security sector institutions remain relevant to global trends and practices. It enables law enforcement agencies in the SADC region to create the necessary leadership and capacity to support governments not only to contain COVID-19 but also in addressing policing challenges that come with natural crises and disasters.

GOVERNMENT'S APPROACH TO SAFETY AND SECURITY GOVERNANCE

The outbreak of COVID-19 in early December 2019 in Wuhan, China, has changed the government's way of dealing with crises and disasters. In particular, the Chinese government and its agencies, including the law enforcement agencies, have transformed China into an effective governance system in terms of managing the COVID-19 pandemic. Global pointers on COVID-19 infections and transmission showed a remarkable decrease in COVID-19 spread in China. World Health Organization's statistics indicate that China managed to contain and reduce COVID-19 infections (WHO, 2020). Comparatively, it appeared that governments in the SADC region were not ready to acknowledge, appreciate, and learn from what the Chinese government has done and achieved; therefore, they were slow in preparing their institutions and making them ready for a possible outbreak of COVID-19 in the region. Four months after the first outbreak of coronavirus in China and the spread of the virus in central Europe, SADC governments were caught heedless and unprepared.

Law enforcement agencies' preparedness and deployment were disappointingly slow in responding to COVID-19. The Namibian government, for example, declared a state of emergency to respond to anticipated national disasters and COVID-19 on March 17, 2020 (Republic of Namibia, 2020), and immediately introduced four stages as a national response to mitigate COVID-19. This was done in terms of article 26 of the Namibian Constitution. In his statement on March 24, 2020, President Geingob warned that "COVID-19 is not only a threat to the lives of the Namibian people and the public health system; it also bears negative economic impacts, threatening the survival of businesses and consequently jobs and livelihoods." The Namibian government eventually declared a lockdown initially in Khomas and Erongo regions on March 27, 2020, when COVID-19 cases stood at eight. Then, the government used the military to erect a COVID-19 emergency facility at Hosea Kutako International Airport, assuming that the airport could be a potential source of COVID-19 spread and infections. This was so because tourists and visitors use Hosea Kutako International Airport as the gate of entry into Namibia. However, four months later, the same facility was relocated to Walvis Bay when the town was declared the epicenter for COVID-19 in Namibia.

On March 15, 2020, President Cyril Ramaphosa declared a state of national disaster in South Africa when the COVID-19 cases stood at 61 and stressed that the COVID-19 pandemic has a "potentially lasting effect" on the country's already slow economic growth. The President revealed the country's [major] concern in dealing with the internal transmission of the virus and that the situation calls for an extraordinary response, saying, "there can be no half measures," (Republic of South Africa, 2020). Other SADC countries, such as Angola, Zambia, and Botswana, have declared a state of emergency to deal with the COVID-19 pandemic. Other SADC governments also followed suit. However, despite resolute decisions taken by SADC governments, the security sector remains poorly prepared and equipped to effectively and efficiently support governments' efforts. The increase in COVID-19 cases in Namibia, Walvis Bay in particular, and in South Africa, Zambia, and Zimbabwe is an indication of poor security sector governance in the SADC region. It is maintained that security sector governance requires coordinated and collaborative efforts. It needs a well-oiled governance system. In summary, effective security sector governance should be an ongoing process that does not start when disaster strikes.

Security sector governance requires sufficient financial resources to be realized. When COVID-19 emerged in the SADC region, governments appeared to gamble for scarce resources (the resources they don't have) to ensure an effective response to the pandemic. The security sector was not prepared. To prevent the spread of COVID-19, it needs a well-funded and coordinated security cluster. The fact is that COVID-19 does not spread through other means than being transported by human beings. In this regard, the manner safety and security institutions manage and conduct their duties has a direct bearing on the spread of the coronavirus. Effective control of the movement of people in the country could limit or delay the infections and eventually the spread of COVID-19. The government needs to provide the necessary support to law enforcement agencies. In the beginning, there have been concerns regarding ill-equipped security sectors in terms of not only well-grounded law enforcement officials but also poorly equipped in terms of personal protective equipment (PPE) to be able to effectively and efficiently perform their constitutional obligations. Therefore, the government approach to security sector governance contributes to effective management and containment of the COVID-19 pandemic.

Another aspect related to security sector governance is the issue of border closures. South Africa's borders were closed on March 15, 2020, after the declaration of a state of national disaster by the President (Republic of South Africa, 2020). While the closure of Namibian borders followed after the declaration of a state of emergency on March 17, 2020 (Republic of South Africa, 2020). These actions were taken four months later, after the first outbreak of COVID-19 in China, and the subsequent spreading of the COVID-19 pandemic in central Europe. The delay in closing the borders in the SADC region might have a hand in the spread of COVID-19 cases. Though it is evident that the index COVID-19 cases in the SADC region were imported, some Namibian and South African borders remained open for "essential services," for example, transportation of essential commodities. Similarly, trans-border activities were also allowed for medical purposes. Interdependence among SADC nations for commodities is a point in question and directly influences governments' decisions and actions regarding trans-border activities. For example, Namibia is dependent on South Africa for essential commodities and medical services. Similarly, Angolan citizens in the southern part of that country are dependent on Namibia for medical treatment and other amenities. The same applies to Botswana/Namibia and

Zambia/Namibia borders. These and other factors forced governments not to entirely close their borders. The aspect of trans-border activities remained a challenge, thereby influencing governments' policies, decisions, and actions and eventually security sector governance. It contributed to a shift in government priorities and actions in slowing down the spreading of COVID-19 to protect people's lives. The protection of human lives has been compromised by economic activities. The call to keep economic activities ongoing to sustain people's livelihoods influences the government's approach to security governance amidst COVID-19.

While trans-border activities continue to be allowed amid the COVID-19 pandemic, control and management of such activities remained a challenge to both governments and law enforcement agencies. Quarantining and testing people involved in trans-border activities remains a daunting task. Law enforcement officials have neither the capacity to be everywhere nor the sufficient resources to escort those people, especially truck drivers, to their destinations to make sure that they do not get in contact with other people. Although no concrete evidence has been brought forward, the perception is that travel-related COVID-19 cases gave rise to increased COVID-19 cases and eventually community transmissions in the SADC region. Therefore, as much as more resources have been committed to COVID-19-related activities such as quarantining suspected people, procuring personal protective equipment, caring for people who contracted the virus, and testing citizens, the same attention has also been focused on security sector governance. The security sector becomes pivotal in the fight against the invisible COVID-19 pandemic. Security governance continues to stretch the government's meager resources and limited efforts; therefore, more needs to be done if COVID-19 is to be effectively and efficiently addressed and contained.

CITIZENS' CIVIC OBLIGATION DURING THE STATE OF EMERGENCY

In a time of national disaster like COVID-19, relevant constitutional provisions may be invoked to obligate government institutions and agencies to act accordingly. Article 26 of the Namibian constitution provides for a declaration of a state of emergency (Republic of Namibia, 1990). Correspondingly, the South African Constitution, article 37, provides for the President to induce the same provision to safeguard the situation (Republic of South Africa, 1996). Similarly, other SADC countries may also invoke their relevant constitutional provisions to protect citizens from deadly and national crises. A state of emergency allows governments to promptly respond and put measures in place to arrest undesirable situations.

The declaration of a state of emergency and a state of national disaster call for citizens' civic responsibility. Citizens are required to abide by the state of emergency regulations to support the government's efforts. In this case, a state of emergency, or state of national disaster, is a situation that calls for both government and citizens' undivided attention and action to ensure that a catastrophic and calamity situation brought on by a sudden outbreak of a disaster like COVID-19 does not restrain the people's livelihoods, health, social, and economic setup and eventually result in loss of lives. In other words, it is a situation that calls for prompt and unreserved action by the government to mitigate the undesired and eruptive situation.

> It is an undeniable fact of life that many states will at some stage be confronted with serious crises, such as wars or other kinds of serious societal upheavals, and that in such situations they may consider it necessary, to restore peace and order, to address public health issues, to limit the enjoyment of individual rights and freedoms and possibly even to suspend their enjoyment altogether. In summary, the government may only succeed if citizens render their undivided attention and collaborative support. (OHCHR 2015, p. 813)

The outbreak of COVID-19 in 2019 has presented exactly the same situation. Globally, governments have declared a state of emergency and locked down their respective countries to enable institutions and agencies to effectively employ measures to protect citizens against the deadly pandemic. Governments in the SADC regions followed suit when the coronavirus walloped their nations in early February 2020. South Africa, Angola, Zambia, Botswana, Zimbabwe, etc. imposed strict state of emergency measures, which became known as "COVID-19 regulations" to guide the operations of the governments in addressing the pandemic.

Namibia introduced four (4) phased stages in March 2020, each with specific but interrelated regulations, to ensure that the government cautiously navigates through the pandemic. Later, in June 2020, a fifth stage was added. Similarly, the South African government followed five (5) phased stages through which the government managed COVID-19. These stiffer measures have resulted in an unbearable situation, not only for people who are affected by COVID-19 and regulations but also for every individual's daily activities and freedom of movement. The resulting restrictions have coerced citizens to comply with the state of emergency regulations. Notwithstanding socioeconomic hardship and unbearable livelihoods, it becomes the civic responsibility of all citizens to demonstrate swiftness in supporting the government to fight and overcome COVID-19. Helao (2015) hypothesizes that the government alone cannot achieve the desired results. It needs cooperation and collaboration by the entire populace. It requires public engagement for law enforcement to succeed. This engagement should be carefully nurtured.

Sigsworth (2019) warns that "public engagement in policing has the potential to develop into an adversarial relationship" if not properly handled. This is essential, especially when society is vulnerable to public health crises such as COVID-19. The health of people becomes the government's biggest priority (Republic of Namibia, 2020; Republic of South Africa, 2020).

Citizens' involvement and support of policing activities are central to police success, especially in times of a state of emergency and national disasters like COVID-19. However, the power accorded to the security sector through COVID-19 regulations may not yield fruit without other sectors' involvement, collaboration, and compliance. Also, in exercising safety and security authority during COVID-19, policing powers should be regulated. Loader (2020) argues that the lockdown [state of emergency] and "its uncertain duration and effects, calls on us to confront some enduring but vital questions about police power and its limits, and about the fragile relationship between the exercise of those powers and public consent" (para.2). Lindblom and Woodhouse (1993) confirmed that to reach a solution without any exercise of power, sheer information and reasoning alone would have to be sufficient to bring all relevant parties into agreement (p. 16).

Helao (2015) put more emphasis on public active participation and compliance with the government's policies. Fundamentally, ever since the inception of formal policing in 1829 in Britain by Sir Robert Peel, the emphasis and focus on citizenry's active participation and their civic obligation toward the security and safety of society have been critical to law enforcement worldwide in reaping benefits to fulfil governmental objectives. Zedner (2006) could not agree more by postulating the fact that there are more talks in police governance literature about "deliberative democracy, participatory democracy, local capacity building and nodal governance all of which claim, in varying degrees, that forms of power-sharing are more effective than top-down instruction" (p. 274).

Scholars like Loader (1997), Hudson (2003), and Johnston and Shearing (2003) also identified and explained major challenges presented by [security] governance as the new sources of security provision, revealing that contemporary policing literature has made a notable contribution to security sector governance, particularly the sectoral approach to resolving policing issues. Therefore, citizens' responsibilities should include aspects of security information sharing, compliance, reporting anti-social behaviors, supporting security and safety initiatives, and significantly holding security sector accountable for their actions. In Namibia, for example, the spike in COVID-19 cases, especially at Walvis Bay and Windhoek, "could have been prevented" (Haufiku, 2020) if a sectoral approach to fighting against the pandemic was adopted. As special advisor to the government on health matters at the time, Dr. Benard Haufiku conceded that the government has failed to coordinate its efforts and bring everyone together, thus losing trust and collaboration in the community and private sector that are critical components in response to COVID-19.

By mid-December 2020, COVID-19 case figures were increasingly terrifying. In the same month, Worldometers (2020) and World Health Organization (2020) provided the following COVID-19 statistics: globally, 71,911,105 cases and 16,08,908 deaths; South Africa, 8,52,965 cases and 23,106 deaths; Zambia, 18,217 cases and 366 deaths; Zimbabwe, 11,219 cases and 307 deaths; Namibia, 16,269 cases and 160 deaths; Angola, 16,061 cases and 365 deaths; and Botswana 12,501 cases and 37 deaths. These figures seem to suggest a second wave of COVID-19, not only in the SADC region but also globally. The above-mentioned figures also show that SADC nations still have a long way to go in terms of arresting the COVID-19 pandemic. In the same vein, it paints a cautionary picture that law enforcement agencies need to step up efforts to strengthen the safety and security of citizens if government objectives to overcome the COVID-19 pandemic are to be realized.

The above figures require governments, private sectors, civic society, and, more importantly, individual citizens to pull efforts together and collaborate to minimize and delay the spread of COVID-19 if the global community is to withstand the deadly pandemic. Citizens' civic obligation and participation are part of security sector governance, which is key to government efforts to fight and suppress global public health crises like COVID-19. The good news is that WHO pins hope on the newly discovered COVID-19 vaccines, which are currently on trial. However, once the effectiveness of those vaccines is successfully confirmed, many countries, especially in the SADC region, may struggle to get access to such vaccines due to financial constraints. Therefore, while nations are awaiting sufficient COVID-19 vaccines to be acquired, law enforcement agencies should not put their feet off the pedal. In summary, cautious and innovative law enforcement should continue even beyond COVID-19.

POST-COVID-19 IMPLICATIONS AND WAY FORWARD

Whereas safety and security sector governance, especially law enforcement, is an unrelenting undertaking, the post-COVID-19 implications for policing should not be overlooked. The COVID-19 pandemic has changed the way police operate, which, to a certain extent, has presented hope and confidence in safety and security governance. However, in the execution of their noble duties, safety and security sector personnel were indiscriminately exposed to the pandemic, and many of them have either succumbed to or been affected by COVID-19. Drew and Martin (2020) noted that

> law enforcement is an occupational group that is more at risk of physical and psychological harm, as its members are called on to be first responders to critical incidents, terrorist attacks, natural disasters, and traumatic events. (p. 31)

Though efforts were redoubled and reinforced during the pandemic to protect both the general public and law enforcement officials, such good efforts and innovative approaches would not stop when the pandemic was over. The efforts and learned best practices would continue. It should be noted that managing crises and pandemics by law enforcement agencies is an opportune learning practices that would shape and benefit safety and security institutions way beyond the COVID-19 pandemic.

Moreover, the innovative way of security sector governance utilized during COVID-19 pandemic has demonstrated that policing institutions can adjust their way of enforcing public health safety regulations and adapt those practices without difficulties. What is important is the general populace's buy-in and cooperation. Therefore, governments should continue sharing accurate COVID-19 data and material support to capacitate law enforcement agencies to prepare and become ready for any resurgence of the pandemic. As discussed in this chapter, the pandemic has allowed safety and security sectors, citizens, and other stakeholders to form a resilient yet mutually collaborative component to manage the pandemic. Essentially, this collaborative effort must constitute a building block toward unremitting future police-community relationships and cooperation if police professionalism is to be maintained and sustained. Gritt and Forsgren (2022) noted that

> COVID-19 has acted as a catalyst for innovation and provided a unique opportunity for the police to identify new workplace learning, for example, what types of innovations worked well, did not work well, and what to carry forward beyond the crisis. (p. 1).

Although the COVID-19 pandemic seems to have subsided, particularly in the SADC region, it is not yet time to take the foot off the pedal. News of the COVID-19 resurgence in Asia should serve as a cautionary wake-up call for the security sector in SADC to continue training and build more capacity to manage both domestic and cross-border situations. It should be noted that the COVID-19 pandemic presented the first health crisis in SADC, which shifted modern-day policing to embrace human compassion more than ever. Law enforcement came out of their "shell" and put on a human face. Police officers have learned that while they are called upon to enforce public health safety measures to protect the general populace, their safety against the COVID-19 pandemic is not guaranteed. Therefore, although the COVID-19 pandemic has created lasting challenges, it has also provided an opportunity for law enforcement to learn, unlearn, and relearn best policing practices.

Gritt and Forsgren (2022) maintained that "the pandemic challenged established assumptions around police work practices and demonstrated that organizational-wide change was possible" (p. 1). In this regard, Gritt and Forsgren added, "the police need to further evaluate its existing assumptions, values, and norms that might limit them to change and transform."

Jones (2020) presented two interesting policing scenario options that would define policing past the COVID-19 pandemic. Firstly, "the police response to the pandemic results in further militarization and draws deeper divides between police and communities" (p. 579), or secondly, "the police response is compassionate and operates procedurally just resulting in the rebuilding of police legitimacy post-pandemic" (p. 579). Given what is discussed in this chapter and Jones' scenario options, the post-COVID-19 implications require a reorganizing and refocusing of learned policing experiences. It is not the purpose of this chapter to discuss Daniel J Jones' two options, but only to cite them to illustrate the potential implications of policing beyond the COVID-19 pandemic. Moving forward, the following are essential:

Embracing best public health safety enforcement practices: Although law enforcement agencies have been prepared to respond to emergencies and crises, the COVID-19 pandemic presented new challenges that resulted in advanced safety and security responses. Some of these practices turned out to be the best policing initiatives that help law enforcement officers successfully manage and contain the situation, hence the need to embrace best policing practices.

Institutionalize innovative policing: Responding to crises and pandemics requires a dedicated safety and security response unit to be established to train and prepare police officers for any contingencies. Emergency management and public health safety measures enforcement go beyond mere policing and need police officers with a human touch to deal with affected communities. Jones (2020) stated that "the police should embrace a guardian mindset during unprecedented and uncertain times" (p. 582) presented by COVID-19. In short, innovative policing should cultivate purposeful capacity and focus, professional approach, learning, and commitment.

Effective partnership and cooperation: Managing the COVID-19 pandemic promotes effective partnership and cooperation, as law enforcement agencies had to mobilize active police-community relationships to manage the pandemic and protect society. This ties in with Jones' second option of "companion and care response when enforcing public health laws due to the pandemic" (p. 579). The approach enhances not only police professionalism but also "police legitimacy" (Jones, 2020, p. 579). The challenge, however, is mobilizing resources to sustain a partnership environment. It requires constant visibility, effective communication, and stakeholder support to manage the police-community partnership.

Strategy excellence and sustainability: Law enforcement operations during COVID-19 pandemic have set a high policing standard and elevated the level of professionalism. As earlier discussed, policing the pandemic has moved the police closer to the people. Whether this approach will continue beyond the pandemic is another question. The approach needs further research and assessment to determine its sustainability. Strategy excellence and sustainability require focused police leadership, material support, and commitment from all stakeholders, and government should play a central role. Therefore, the post-COVID-19 implications pose surmountable challenges to the safety and security sectors. Learning the best policing strategies should continue to build law enforcement capacity going forward.

CONCLUSION

COVID-19 cases and their devastating effects are raging globally, regionally, and domestically; thus, intensified efforts are needed to safeguard humanity. Security sector governance and the manner law enforcement dealt with the COVID-19 pandemic in the SADC region vary due to socioenvironment and available resources. In essence, security sector's preparedness and readiness came under scrutiny, especially from the citizens' side. For the first time, it turned out to be a naked reality that the government's approach to governance and service provision in terms of advancing socioeconomic and people's livelihoods have an impact on efforts to contain domestic crises and disasters such as COVID-19. In reality, the spreading of the COVID-19 pandemic cannot be arrested in a society that is succumbing to countless socioeconomic challenges, for example, poverty, unemployment, poor social safety nets, etc.

The aforementioned issues, to a certain degree, have contributed to non-compliance with the state of emergency regulations, therefore rendering both citizens' civic obligations and the security sector's duties and responsibilities ineffective. Besides, the government's approach to public sector governance has complicated the whole aspect of managing public health crises to arrest the COVID-19 infection rate. Poor housing, water scarcity, and poor infrastructure undermine the security sector's capacity to mitigate the deadly coronavirus. Law enforcement agencies found themselves in a peculiar situation.

Also, the lack of transport to access all corners and reach every village in the country, and the fact that they were also poorly equipped in terms of personal protective equipment, are added challenges to already poor-resourced security sectors. Therefore, governments like those in Namibia and South Africa turned to the International Monetary Fund (IMF) for financial assistance to fund COVID-19-related activities. Certainly, COVID-19 serves as a lesson and learning experience for SADC governments to realign their structures and efforts in terms of governance and prepare themselves for future public health crises. In the same vein, security sector institutions, particularly law enforcement agencies, should train and develop their personnel and prepare them to be able to support government efforts during state of emergency and national disasters. The COVID-19 pandemic may not end anytime soon. Also, governments are likely to open up to revive the economic sector. This will place added challenges on sectors that are tasked with COVID-19 responsibility, which in the end will raise the pandemic curve. Finally, the proposed COVID-19 vaccine, though not discussed in this chapter, should be approached with caution. In the meantime, the enforcement of COVID-19 measures by law enforcement agencies must continue. Law enforcement agencies should embrace best practices and experiences learned during COVID-19 to enhance capacity going forward. Post-COVID-19 ramifications, as discussed in this chapter, call for innovative and focused police leadership to direct enforcement of future crises and state of emergency regulations, particularly in SADC region.

REFERENCES

Abnöther, A. H., Fluri, P. H., & Jurekovic, P. (Eds). *Security Sector Governance in the Western Balkans: Self-Assessment Studies on Defence, Intelligence, Police and Border Management Reform.* Vienna and Geneva, 2007.

Bittner, E. The Police on Skid-row: A Study of Peace Keeping. *American Sociology Review*, 32(5), (1967), 669–715. https://doi:10.2307/2092019

Bratianu, C. Organizational Learning and the Learning Organization. (2015). Retrieved from https://www.researchgate.net/publication/322235340_Organizational_Learning_and_the_Learning_Organization

Bruce, D. Covid-19: Police Abuse of Powers Reveals Systematic Flaws. *Mail & Guardian* (16 April 2020).

Burger, J. Preparation is Key to Policing a Crisis like Covid-19. Institute of Security Studies. (2020, April 20). Retrieved from https://issafrica.org/iss.today/preparations-is-key-to-policing-a-crisis-like-Covid-19

Drew, J. M. & Martin, S. Mental Health and Well-Being of Police in a Health Pandemic: Critical Issues for Police Leaders in a Post-covid-19 Environment. *Journal of Community Safety and Well-Being*, 5(2), (2020), 31–36.

Engel, R. S., Cosaro, N., & Ozser, M. M. The Impact of Police on Criminal Justice Reform: Evidence from Cincinnati, Ohio. *Criminology and Public Policy*, 10(16), (2017), 375–402. https://doi.org/10.1111/1745-9133.12299

Graduate Institute Geneva & Global Health Centre. *Policy Brief: The Security Sector and Global Health Crises: Lessons and Prospects*. DCAF (2015).

Gritt, E. & Forsgren, E. *Policing in a Hybrid Work Environment: Challenges and Lessons Learned, Adapatation, Information Management Technology,* March 2022Retrieved from: https//business.leeds.ac.uk/research-aimtech/dir-record/research-blog/1961/policing-in-a-hybrid-work-environment-challenges-and-l.

Haufiku, B. We Could Have Prevented This. *Windhoek Observer* (2020, July 22).

Helao, T. *An Evaluation of Good Governance and Service Delivery at Sub-National Levels in Namibia: The Case of the Oshana Region.* Pretoria: University of South Africa (2015).

Hoogenwoning, F. C. *The Police Evolution: Vision on Policing.* Project Group Vision on Policing. The Hague: Dutch National Police Institute (2006).

Hudson, B. *Justice in the Risk Society.* London: Sage (2003).

Hylton, R. *Law Enforcement Role in Responding to Disasters.* Washington: FEMA (2013).

INTERPOL. *Covid-19 Pandemic: Guidelines for Law Enforcement* (26 March 2020). Retrieved from www.Covid-19_LE_Guidelines_PUBLIC_26march2020.pdf

Johnston, L. & Shearing, C. *Governing Security: Explorations in Policing and Justice.* London: Routledge (2003).

Jones, D. J. The Potential Impacts of Pandemic Policing on Police Legitimacy: Planning Past the Covid-19 Crisis. *Policing: A Journal of Policy and Practice*, 14(3), (2020), 579–586.

Kavari, M. Policing towards 4th Industrial Revolution in the Namibian Context. *Namibian Police Journal*, Issue 2 (2 May 2020).

Kelling, G. L. Police and Communities: The Quiet Revolution. *Perspectives on Policing*, 1(June), (1988), 1–8.

Lindblom, C. E. & Woodhouse, E. J. *The Policy-Making Process,* 3rd edition. New Jersey: Upper Saddle River (1993).

Loader, I. Coronavirus: Why We Must Tackle Hard Questions about Police Power. Oxford University (2020). Retrieved from https://law.ox.uk/news.2020.-04-16-policing-covid-19.crisis

Loader, I. Plural Policing and Democratic Governance. *Social Legal Studies*, 9, (2000), 323.

Loader, I. & Walker, N. Policing as a Public Good: Reconstituting the Connections between Policing and the State. *Theoretical Criminology*, 5(1), (2001), 9–35.

Luscombe, A. & McClelland, A. *Policing the Pandemic: Tracking the Policing of Covid-19 across Canada.* White paper (9 April 2020). Retrieved from www.policing_the_pandemic_white_paper_9April2020.pdf

Masake, P. H. *A Critical Consideration of the Exclusion of Corporate Criminal Liability for the Atrocity Crimes under the Rome Statute of the International Criminal Court.* South Africa: University of Stellenbosch (2019).

May, P. J. & Williams, W. *Disaster Policy Implementation: Managing Programmes under Shared Governance.* New York: Plenum (1986).

Ngoma, N. *Prospects for a Security Community in Southern Africa: An Analysis of Regional Security in the Southern African Development Community.* Pretoria: Institute for Security Studies (2005).

Office of High Commission for Human Rights. *Human Rights in the Administration of Justice: A Manual on Human Rights for Judges, Prosecutors and Lawyers.* Professional training series no. 9. New York: United Nations (2003). Retrieved from https://www.ohchr.org/Documents/Publications/training9Titleen.pdf

Rauch, J. Police Reform and South Africa's Transition. Paper presented at the *South African Institute for International Affairs* conference (2000). Centre for the study of violence and reconciliation.

Republic of Namibia. Briefing Statements by His Excellency the President, Dr. Hage, G. Geingob on Covid-19 National Response Measures. (March 2020). Windhoek.

Republic of Namibia. *Police Act 1990* (Act 19 of 1990). Ministry of Justice: Government Printers.

Republic of Namibia. Opening Statement by His Excellency the President, Dr. Hage, G Geingob at the Media Briefing on Regulations for the Covid-19 Khomas and Erongo Lockdown. (27 March 2020).

Republic of Namibia. *The Constitution of the Republic of Namibia*. Ministry of Justice: Government Printers (1990).

Republic of South Africa. *Declaration of State of Emergency: National Disaster (COVID-19)*. Published in Government Gazette no. 7148 on 18 March 2020, Proclamation 7 of 2020 (2020).

Republic of South Africa. *South African Police Service Act, 1995 (Act 68 of 1995)*. Ministry of Justice: Government Printers.

Republic of South Africa. *The Constitution of the Republic of South Africa*. Pretoria: Government Printers.

Ruppel, O. C. Regional Economic Communities and Human Rights in East and Southern Africa. In Bosl, A. & Diescho, J. (eds.), *Human Rights in Africa: Legal Perspectives on their Protection and Promotion*. Namibia: Macmillan (2009).

Sigsworth, R. *Harnessing Public Engagement for Police Accountability in Africa*. Africa Report 21. Institute for Security Studies (2019).

Sorensen, J. S. & Soderbaum, F. The End of the Development-Security Nexus: The Rise of Global Disaster Management. Uppsala: Dag Hammarskjold. *Development dialogue, No.* (58 April 2012).

Wood, J. D. Pioneers of Policing: Clifford Shearing. (2014). Retrieved from https://doi.org/10.1080/15614263.2014.893967. pp. 519–532.

World Health Organization. *Emergencies, Preparedness and Response: Disaster Outbreak News*. (2019). Retrieved from https://www.who.int/csr/don/12-january-2020-novel-coronavirus-china/en/

World Health Organization. *The Health of the People, What Works: The African Regional Health Report 2014*. Brazzaville: WHO Regional Office for Africa (2014).

World Health Organization. *WHO Coronavirus (Covid-19) Dashboard*. (2020). Retrieved from https://covid19.who.int/?gclid=CjwKCAjwmrn5BRB2EiwAZgL9okdksfc7TV6BWZIjexSMcbERZuUhF7pgknFzOWG3rrh7DjqKqcMTAhoCo6oQAvD_BwE

Worldometers. Covid-19 Coronavirus Statistics. (2020). Retrieved from https://www.worldometers.info/coronavirus/

Zedner, L. *Liquid Security: Managing the Market for Crime Control*. UK: University of Oxford (2006).

Chapter 6

The Impact of COVID-19 Policies on Survival Immigrants

The Botswana and South African Response

Mbetu Gamuchirai and Masake Pilisano Harris

INTRODUCTION

The rapid spread of the COVID-19 pandemic left many governments unable to clearly map a way forward for operations in their countries without infringing on many of their inhabitants' rights. Worldwide governments had to make decisions and weigh equally, important values: protect people from COVID-19, on one end, and on the other end, limit certain rights to contain the virus and slow down its spread. Generally, the consensus across the world was to instill lockdowns in their countries.

Prior to the COVID-19 era, the term lockdown was reserved for confined spaces such as prisons or schools for the prevention of an outbreak of violence or disease (Nolan, 2011, p. 169). A lockdown may be called by administrative officials, law enforcement agencies, or other emergency responders. The lockdown included the limitation of travel beyond one's province. Lockdowns in most countries also involved the complete shutdown of borders and restrictions on travel. There were special permissions for repatriated citizens who would be allowed to move into and out of countries under special conditions. This brought legal intra-border trading to a halt and had devastating effects within trade blocs, whereby permits and quarantine conditions were now required to transport goods. For individual, cross-border traders, the consequences were dire in that some were stuck in the country in which they purchased the goods but were unable to return home to sell said goods. Or were in their home country and unable to purchase goods across the border.

African governments have always struggled with integrating the informal sector into the mainstream economy; however, the impact of this sector on the economy became glaring during the lockdown. For example, in South Africa and Zimbabwe, numerous complaints arose, with people arguing that staying at home would lead to starvation and that they would rather face the consequences of COVID-19 than watch their family members starve (Voice of America, 2020).

Some countries initiated different levels of lockdowns, which included absolutely no movement beyond your residence and individuals could only move if they had a permit that would allow them to either go to work, buy food, or exercise. In certain countries, there was a reduction in the workforce, where only essential workers were allowed to work during lockdowns. This group of people was known as Essential Critical Infrastructure Workers. The Center for Disease Control and Prevention (CDC, 2020), USA, defines this group as being:

> Functioning critical infrastructure is imperative during the response to the Covid 19 emergency for both public health and safety as well as community well-being. Certain critical infrastructure industries have a special responsibility in these times to continue operations. (CDC, 2020)

These essential industries were allowed to function with special permissions. Even within those industries, there was a maximum percentage. However, most of the workforce was expected to remain at home. The effect included that the employers were unable to pay their employees, and many had to retrench workers or stop hiring casual workers. Although some governments were able to initiate stipends for small and medium enterprises (SMEs) and a subsistence allowance, these were usually only considered for registered SMEs with legitimate employees. Legitimate employees are those who are in South Africa legally and have the requisite paperwork to hold employment with the relevant social security numbers. Non-citizens were, at large excluded, from government stipends.

One of the consequences of this policy in South Africa and Botswana was that many illegitimate workers from their neighboring country, Zimbabwe, were stranded without a source of income. Unsurprisingly, many Zimbabweans who had fled the flailing economy of their own country found themselves stranded and desperate. Reports in newspapers in South Africa and Botswana found that many Zimbabweans were approaching the police stations to be repatriated to their home country as they could not survive in the state of lockdown. In some countries, lockdowns lasted for over three months, with only some industries, such as retail stores, mining, and restaurants, opening when the lockdowns were lifted.

The following section provides a definition of survival immigration, the tenets of the lockdown, the laws that were initiated as a result, and the short- and long-term consequences of immigrant status, with a particular focus on survival immigrants.

WHAT IS A SURVIVAL MIGRANT?

The term "survival migrant" is recognizable by its name, that is, immigrants who migrate for the purposes of survival. Although it may appear obvious, public international law is oblivious to this group of people. In the absence of migration and trade agreements between countries to address the needs of the survival immigrants, the survival immigrants are left to their own devices, as they do not qualify as refugees (Betts, 2013). The distinction that Betts draws between survival immigrants and refugees is that refugees are trying to flee persecution while survival migrants are "fleeing other sources of serious human rights deprivations" (Betts, 2013). Article 1 of the 1951 Refugee Convention defines refugees as:

> Someone who is unable or unwilling to return to their country of origin owing to a well-founded fear of being persecuted for reasons of race, religion, nationality, membership of a particular social group, or political opinion.

It is commendable that there is an international framework dedicated to the receipt of refugees that nations can assent to and perform some reciprocity by taking in refugees. Internationally, countries take over the social protection role that the originating country can no longer provide. The treaty of the 1951 Refugee Convention is based on the underlying principle of *non-refoulement.* This principle entails that a refugee cannot be returned to his/her originating country where he/she will suffer further persecution. However, certain countries may try to reduce their obligations, costs, and influx of refugees by limiting the definition of refugees or asylum seekers. Giesel (2019) argues that the limitation of the definition is encouraged by how the Refugee Convention is not strictly applied. Countries, therefore, have agency over the definition. Furthermore, a country may create other policies that limit the entry of refugees or movement within the state.

South Africa recently amended its Refugee Act to limit the rights of refugees in their country. The limitations include not being able to participate in political activity in their country of birth or the prevention of applying for refugee status if they arrived in South Africa illegally. Even seeking public services in their originating country may lead to the removal of their refugee status. An asylum seeker does not have automatic rights to study or work in South Africa and requires further permissions. The system has become so restrictive that people coming from surrounding countries would rather live in foreign countries without legal status. It has been argued that although this is contrary to the *non-refoulement* principle, with increasing poverty and unemployment levels, South Africa has had to increase its social protection budget on average by 7.9 percent annually (Mtantato, 2018). This, of course, is expected to have increased more in 2020 during the COVID-19 pandemic to support the worsening social protection burden. The social protection budget is likely to prioritize its citizens, which further marginalizes refugees. The effect is to encourage refugees to be more dependent on donor intervention.

The Botswana Refugee (Recognition and Control) Act of 1968 is stricter than its neighbor's. It restricts movement from refugee camps created for the purposes of holding refugees. Botswana recognizes political refugees despite not having a clear definition of what a political refugee is, as this remains at the discretion of the Minister of Immigration in terms of the Refugee (Recognition and Control) Act of 1968. Botswana has similar legal structures to South Africa in that political refugees are not allowed to participate in any other politics in Botswana or any other country, including their original country. In this regard, the status of refugees is limited, leaving those who are fleeing their countries in a state without real status or agency. The legitimate route to come in as a skilled laborer is quite cumbersome, as employers must prove why an immigrant person must be employed instead of an indigenous person/citizen. It must also be shown that there are no local candidates for this role. Those with minimal skills and education are left out of the option of legitimate migration. Thus, leaving a gap wherein survival immigrants are unable to legitimize their immigration status (Polus, 2012).

Botswana has been recognized as having a strict policy on refugees and not accepting economic refugees. Once one is on the fringe, they are excluded from accessing health services for chronic care such as HIV care and treatment, as well as treatment for other chronic diseases such as cancer. Without paperwork, one is subject to immediate arrest and deportation. Many Zimbabweans, Mozambicans, and Malawians live as illegal immigrants to make ends meet with menial jobs and casual work that does not require documentation. A key aspect of being a survival migrant is one's obligation to remit a significant portion of one's earnings to their family back home, leaving them with minimal savings. Their home countries thus benefit from foreign remittances as well as their host country (Slay & Peleah, 2015).

As there is no clear international legal framework for survival migrants, this group of people will largely become illegal immigrants unless amnesty is granted. Survival immigrants are known to come from fragile states where persecution is not blatant in the absence of a civil war. However, human rights violations in their home countries are rampant. Betts (2013) states that the greatest problem with survival migration is that the definition is not set and are thus likely to be left without a secure legal migration status. Sometimes countries extend the definition of refugees to include survival migrants, but their inclusion is inconsistent in different jurisdictions. Immigrants from Malawi and Zimbabwe may not necessarily be persecuted in their homelands. However, they are unable to attain sustainable livelihoods in their countries because they are subject to extreme poverty. In addition, these migrants may be fleeing political oppression stemming from unfavorable policies and practices that are synonymous with fragile states. Since these reasons do not fit squarely into any definition for the purposes of legal migration, Survival Immigrants may include those who: arrived within the receiving countries on legitimate visas that have lapsed; may have crossed the borders illegally; or may have forged paperwork (Betts, 2013).

The livelihoods of survival immigrants remain a contentious issue as they operate economically outside of the law and cannot seek recourse from it. That is, while they are in foreign countries and are undocumented, they cannot look to the police if they are disenfranchised. Further, they are unable to gain access to social welfare services such as discounted health care services or schooling for their children. Survival migrants must live with a minimal digital footprint to avoid attracting attention to themselves. This includes getting casual jobs that pay in cash and are usually based on verbal contracts. Such contracts can be unilaterally broken by the employer with minimal consequences. Disputes with employers may result in deportation; as such, they cannot grow beyond unskilled jobs or elementary occupations. Elementary occupations are noted by the International Labor Organization (ILO) as "consisting of simple and routine tasks which mainly require the use of hand-held tools and often some physical effort" (ILO, 2004).

These are ongoing problems that continue to manifest as states within the Southern African Development Community (SADC) become more fragile and the immigration policies in the abovenamed countries remain the same. Studies have been conducted to determine the extent of the contribution of the survival migrants to the economies that they reside in; however, the data remains based on approximations as they are largely an invisible group. A primary example would be in South Africa, where an estimated 1.5 million Zimbabweans reside and about 50 percent of them are undocumented (Truen, 2016). The extent of this lack of documentation has led to the South African government granting amnesties to undocumented Zimbabweans to alleviate the cumbersome deportation process overwhelming the South African Ministry of Home Affairs (Khumalo, 2014). The last amnesty in South Africa was in 2014, when 300,000 Zimbabweans were granted residency through the Zimbabwe Special Dispensation Permit (ZSP). Another such amnesty was granted in 2009, whereby Zimbabweans were granted the opportunity to legitimize their stay for the purposes of work or study (Goitom, 2017). The ZSP was extended for another 3 years in 2017, under the name Zimbabwe Exemption permit (ZEP) which was set to expire in December 2021 (Schensema, 2023). The Department of Home

Affairs (DHA) on 29 November 2021 announced that the permit would not be extended. ZEP holders were given 12 months until December 2022 to apply for alternative immigration status. A further 6 months until June 2023 was given. However the High Court of South Africa overturned the DHA's decision to cancel such permits as there was no consultation process, thereby making the decision unlawful (The Associated Press, 2023).

Botswana has had no such amnesty to date. According to Voice of America (2019), Botswana spends approximately USD 100,000.00 per annum deporting Zimbabweans (Dube, 2019). The strict policy dictates that if one is found without paperwork, they are immediately arrested and deported. In 2008, it was estimated that approximately one million Zimbabweans crossed the border into Botswana, with about 100,000 Zimbabwean immigrants still living in Botswana (Betts, 2013). Approximately 40,000 Zimbabweans are thought to be illegal immigrants who work in domestic work, vending, farm work, construction, and other menial work.

The number of Zimbabwean deportees has steadily increased. It is unclear if this is a signal of an increase in Zimbabwean immigrants or a stricter immigration policy. However, the Botswana Government uses a significant amount of its resources to deport survival migrants. By virtue of their illegal immigration status and types of employment survival, migrants are less likely to be present in the employment records of employers. Some attempts to detect this group would be using the statistics of people who enter the country with temporary visas and then never return even after their visas efflux. Migrants within this group are more likely to be seen as invisible contributors, where survival migrants are noted as employees but are not registered with any other official body, such as a trade union or social protection agency. An Organization for Economic Co-operation and Development (OECD) and International Labor Organization (ILO) (2018) study showed the contribution of immigrants disaggregated by race. It was found that generally black immigrants in South Africa were overrepresented in the following categories: service, shop, and market sales workers; legislators, senior officials, and management; craft-related trades workers; and elementary workers. Although there are some less vulnerable types of jobs, it can be noted that those jobs are reserved for legitimate migrants and not survival immigrants.

The OECD/ILO (2018) study reflects that generally immigrants have a positive impact on the society as it reflects an increase in the supply of differently skilled labor. The counterargument in this regard is that the role of the receiving country is to be prepared or have immigration policies that are focused on economic growth. Essentially, space must be created for immigrants to participate and contribute to the development of the country. In the South African context, the inclusion of immigrants has shown that immigrants contribute to an increase in Gross Domestic Product (GDP) per capita as they are able to integrate well into economy and drive productivity. It has been discovered that during 2001 and 2011, foreign-born employees paid more income tax than native-born South Africans, and they spent significantly less of the public expenditure than native-born South Africans (OECD/ ILO, 2018). One could deduce that if survival migrants were given legal status, their contribution would be significant. Unfortunately, in the absence of data confirming this contribution, survival migrants can be easily dismissed as a burden despite their contribution to the economy. The result of their invisibility was especially highlighted during the COVID-19 pandemic, where survival migrants were excluded from accessing welfare grants.

COVID-19 LAWS

The South African shut down was instituted at levels from 1 to 5. Some companies, if their type of work allowed, opted to have their staff work remotely. Remote working was not a practical option for retail and the service industry, such as restaurants, domestic work, and farm work, where there is a higher proportion of employees who are survival migrants. Certain industries, such as fast food and fine dining outlets, most retail stores, and beauty industry, had to shut down completely and await the normalization of business activities (Russ, 2020).

To affect the relevant laws during this period, the President declared a state of National Disaster in March 2020. A state of National Disaster allowed for the creation of laws in response to the COVID-19 pandemic, which had an overall effect on a significant number of existing regulations. Laws particularly affecting human rights, working conditions, civil and religious participation, and the economy were impacted. The National Disaster of note was the rate at which the disease was spreading and South Africa's health systems' limited capacity to manage the dire consequences of the spread of the disease. Having noted the experience in Italy, the United Kingdom, and China, South Africa was quick to limit movement in and out of the country (Reyburn, 2020). All international passenger flights were banned except for repatriation purposes or with special permission from the Minister of Transport. Cross-border passenger transport was effectively banned for the duration of the lockdown and state of emergency, except for purposes of repatriation in terms of directions issued in regulations made under Section 27 (2) of the National Disaster Management Act (Act 57 of 2002).

The Botswana government made the decision to close all its borders on March 28, 2020. The closure of borders came after one COVID-19 fatality. Any cross-border travel was limited to essential services. Soon after, a state of emergency was declared on March 31, 2020, and came into effect on April 2, 2020. Like in South Africa, a lockdown was instituted ranging from levels 1 to 4 in Botswana. In the same fashion, the higher the level of lockdown, the greater the restrictions on business and movement. All public transport was banned except for purposes of repatriation and the movement of essential goods and services. Again, the service and retail industries suffered the most as their clientele could not access them. The national legislature implemented a national state of emergency, which included giving all the legislative power to the President to allow him to make changes or amendments to the law without having to take the normal legislative route for law creation during the state of National Disaster in terms of the Disaster Management Act, 2002.

To support small and medium enterprises that were struggling, the South African and Botswana governments resolved to provide relief funds for businesses to allow them to continue to pay their employees. Companies had to downsize to be able to make up for the absence of business during extended lockdowns. New labor laws that were added allowed the state to provide an unemployment benefit to employees that may have been on casual or wage contracts who were now without income. Such benefits in both countries were issued from a relief fund that was created from the government emergency fund, taxes, and the donations of well-wishers.

The closure of borders had implications for survival immigrants who are cross-border traders and those who are dependent on the service industry for casual work. Because the economies in Botswana and South Africa were closed, this population was now stuck in foreign lands without income or means of survival. As already noted, survival migrants in this context are usually in jobs where the income is enough for sustenance rather than being a long-term source of wealth. Such informal arrangements are likely to mean a lack of access to formal wealth or savings mechanisms such as a bank account. As such, the consequences of a lockdown are dire and further disenfranchise this group, whose families are sustained mainly through their remittances to their home countries (Chami, 2020).

In the South African context, the Minister of Employment and Labor Affairs released a law introducing the COVID-19 scheme. As empowered by Regulation 10 (8) of the Regulations issued by the Minister of Cooperative Governance and Traditional Affairs in terms of section 27 (2) of the Disaster Management Act, 2002 (Act No. 57 of 2002). The COVID-19 relief scheme included the term "temporary layoff." A temporary layoff was explained as a reduction in the workforce resulting from the closure of business operations completely or temporarily during the period of National Disaster. In South African law, the term "temporary layoff" was preferable during the COVID-19 pandemic to avoid mass retrenchments and the costs thereof. It allowed employers to terminate employment for the duration of the lockdown and then re-employ employees after lockdown when businesses resumed. The temporary layoff option unfortunately was not conducive for many employees, as they were not entitled to a wage during the lay-off period. Of course, it was highly likely that management would prefer to lay off employees who were working entry-level jobs and performing unskilled labor. These groups of employees are more likely to be hired under informal arrangements and are more expendable to the business. Such informal arrangements usually include undocumented survival immigrants.

Notice 215 of the Department of Labor in South Africa gave birth to the COVID-19 Temporary Employee/Employer Relief Scheme. The Employee/Employer Relief Scheme was established to alleviate the economic impact of COVID-19. This notice made provision for both employers and employees to apply for a grant during the COVID-19 lockdown. This scheme was reserved for employers who, because of the COVID-19 pandemic, had to close their operations for three (3) months or a lesser period and would suffer financial distress. The payments from this scheme were delinked from the normal Unemployment Insurance Fund (UIF). That is, this particular benefit only paid for the cost of salaries for employees during the temporary closure of business. This UIF benefit was capped at a maximum level of R17,712.00 per month per employee and was to be paid on a sliding scale, with an income replacement rate of 38 percent to 60 percent. Such payment was mandated to be maintained at least at par with the sector-specific minimum wage. An illness benefit was also included for employees on 14-day quarantine as per Notice 215 of the Department of Labor in South Africa.

Despite the availability of such a safety net for approximately 11 million employees in the formal sector, only 55,268 applications had been processed by April 20, 2020 (Runciman, 2020). This result on its own is not conclusive, as there are a plethora of reasons why more companies would not have accessed this benefit. Such reasons include that companies may have had the means to continue operating, while others did not have the means, care, or understanding of the COVID-19 temporary relief scheme. The relief scheme also excluded approximately 3 million workers employed in the informal sector, where most of the survival migrants belong. In some instances, employers were said to be applying the no work, no pay principle, which, as implied, means that if one is not physically present at work, one should not expect to receive any wages (Kavuro, 2020). Additionally, employers who did not contribute to the UIF were initially excluded as beneficiaries, thereby also depriving their employees of relief during the lockdown. However, such unregistered employers were empowered through this scheme to approach the UIF directly to claim relief, but they were required to register first. In some instances the system that would disallow online registration for UIF, but one could physically register at their offices. However, the queues were long, and social distancing could not be properly implemented in those queues (Kavuro, 2020). Furthermore, such registration would have excluded undocumented survival immigrants who were formally employed.

Another relief scheme named the Social Distress Grant, which provided a stipend of R350 per month, was available in South Africa during the early COVID-19 era. According to Kavuro (2020), for someone to qualify, they were expected to fulfil the following criteria:

- Be a South African citizen, permanent resident, or a refugee registered with Home Affairs;
- Reside within the borders of the Republic of South Africa;
- Above the age of 18;
- Unemployed;
- Not receiving any income;
- Not receiving any social grants;
- Not receiving any unemployment insurance benefit and does not qualify to receive unemployment insurance benefits;
- Not receiving a stipend from the National Student Financial Aid Scheme;
- Not receiving any other government COVID-19 response support; and
- Not resident of a government-funded or subsidized institution.

Survival migrants were immediately disqualified for their illegitimate residency in South Africa. The rest of the requirements became redundant in the absence of legal status. Therefore, the COVID-19-related policies created a crisis for survival migrants and highlighted the glaring ignorance of the contribution of this population to the economy. However, immigrants whose paperwork had expired during lockdown were automatically granted an extension until July 31, 2020. In response to the COVID-19 lockdown of industries, the Botswana government developed a COVID-19 Wage Fund for employees and employers.

The employee subsidy would be 50 percent of a wage of at least BWP 1,500.00 and not more than BWP 2,500.00. Like the South African experience, the wage subsidy was reserved for Botswana citizens. Unlike South Africa, Botswana excluded immigrants with permanent residence or refugee status. The social relief fund also included food hampers for vulnerable people who must also have been citizens. The COVID-19 Relief Fund of Botswana was made up of donations and government funds. Despite tax contributions from non-citizens as legitimate workers or otherwise, they did not have access to the relief fund. Low-income migrants had to depend on donations from well-wishers. An organization called Sisonke identified 800 sex workers who required food assistance, the majority of whom are migrants to whom they made food donations (Dube, 2020). The target population or criteria for this donor providing COVID-19 relief were: sex workers who were HIV positive, had children, and were foreigners. This reiterates that there were gaps in population coverage due to the social welfare grant, as there are many vulnerable groups that could have been included (Dube, 2020).

During the lockdown, illegal immigrants were granted amnesty by allowing them to stay in Botswana undocumented. This was due to the immigration offices being closed and largely overwhelmed by the influx of extension applications, as migrants could no longer cross the border to renew their permit, and returning to their home countries would mean they would be subjected to quarantine in sometimes questionable facilities. In Malawi, 400 people who had been deported from South Africa fled a quarantine site because of the poor living conditions; the facilities allegedly did not have water, food, or sanitation (Ankara, 2020). Additionally, quarantine in some countries was done at a personal cost that many migrants would not have been able to afford. Survival migrants were further marginalized during the COVID-19 era. Without legitimate employment, they also would not have a legitimate means of claiming anything against an employer if their contracts were terminated.

The Impact of COVID-19

As noted above, COVID-19 gave survival migrants some element of legitimacy as they were allowed to stay in foreign countries during the lockdown. However, this legitimacy was only for the duration of the lockdown. After the second lockdown, migrants seeking extensions were instructed to return as the borders were now open for repatriation purposes in South Africa and Botswana. Moreover, the amnesty was not necessarily beneficial to migrants if they were unable to derive income during this period, as most industries were closed. In South Africa, asylum seekers whose asylum had expired during lockdown and were unable to renew during this time had their bank accounts frozen and were unable to access funds (Rugunanan, 2020). Asylum seekers who had legitimate status were therefore lumped together with survival migrants and could not access the unemployment fund.

One of the most detrimental impacts was the lack of income and poverty, to the extent that some survival migrants were approaching the police for deportation. In April 2020 alone, in Botswana, 500 Zimbabweans were deported who had approached the state for help to return to their home country, as they were impoverished (Mosikare, 2020). In an act of desperation, migrants approached authorities, stating that they would much rather be deported than continue to live in the dire conditions of poverty that they were currently living under. In South Africa, 439 Mozambicans, 538 Zimbabweans, and hundreds of Malawians and Zambians were deported between April and May 2020 (Mosikare, 2020).

Access to Health Care

Access to health care is a universal right that is enshrined in both the South African and Botswana Constitutions. South Africa has a generally open health care system that provides access to all human beings, regardless of immigration status, for free at point of care. Contrastingly, Botswana only provides free health care to its citizenry; foreigners must pay additional amounts, although healthcare is subsidized. Studies have noted that migrants who are generally more vulnerable to diseases are more likely to have limited access to healthcare. This is especially visible within the COVID-19 context of the crisis, where coping mechanisms like returning to their home countries for treatment were not plausible.

During the pandemic, survival migrants were not only deprived of economic income; they were also deprived of access to free health care services. In the South African context, to access free health services and be tested for COVID-19, one had to present identification of either a South African Identification Card or passport, which would be screened for the purposes of legitimacy. Survival immigrants who are without proper paperwork were likely deterred from seeking these services to avoid deportation. Concerns were noted in that information on testing and screening is to be kept for six weeks after the end of the state of emergency. There was a lingering fear that such information may be used to identify illegal migrants and lead to their arrest and deportation. Normally, refugees and asylum seekers, with or without permits, can access health care for free of charge at point of care (Scalabrini, 2020). Accessing health care would not impact their immigrant status.

The Botswana health care system has always been clear that its health care system is reserved for its citizenry. Permanent residents have access to medical aid or the option to pay cash for medical services. A detrimental aspect of this is that survival migrants are less likely to seek medical attention even in the face of being exposed to COVID-19, as it is expensive and threatens to expose their illegal status. Another glaring issue for survival migrants is the lack of free access to anti-retroviral treatment (ART) for the treatment of HIV. The policy on this has been clear in that migrants are excluded from accessing ART for free in Botswana. Some Zimbabwean migrants would arrange for a runner or, in their own, capacity register for ART in the border towns in Zimbabwe and periodically collect from the border towns. During lockdown, this was no longer an option, which led to significant defaults on treatment. Studies have shown that one of the inhibitors of success in getting 95 percent of people tested, treated, and their viral loads repressed in Botswana to reach the 95-95-95 targets is the lack of access to ART for migrants (Carter, 2020).

LATENT ISSUES CONCERNING SURVIVAL IMMIGRANTS AND POST-COVID-19 IMPLICATIONS

The Recognition of Human Rights

One of the things conflated by the COVID-19 pandemic is the failure to recognize the human rights of survival and/or undocumented migrants. Moyo and Zanker (2022) recognize this as a purposeful attempt by the South African immigration system to mostly exclude other Africans, especially survival migrants, from attaining any legitimacy. This unfortunately manifests as xenophobia at grassroot level within communities. The COVID-19 situation highlighted complicated and ever-changing legislative systems that tend to segregate labor immigrants and exclude survival migrants completely from the system. Such segregation occurs in separating asylum seekers according to their labor skills, which in some contexts could be determined as granting them status not provided to survival migrants. A key moment proving this segregation was during one of the immigration amnesties conducted by the South African government, wherein 45,255 people abandoned their asylum seeker claims in pursuit of alternative residential status (Moyo & Zanker, 2022). Thereby, suggesting that a significant number of asylum seekers are also survival migrants who are attempting to legitimize their legal status in the country as labor migrants.

Political Rhetoric and the Human Rights of Civil Servants

The political rhetoric surrounding immigrants generally has impacted survival, severely leading to xenophobic attacks during and after COVID-19 lockdowns in South Africa. The political rhetoric included defining survival immigrants without sufficient paperwork as criminals who deserved any xenophobic attacks despite their contributions to the informal economy. There is also continued discussion of them being a burden on the health care system, thereby displacing citizens from accessing social welfare services and employment. Maphosa and Ntau (2021) identify undocumented immigrants in South Africa and Botswana as "*Homo Sacer,*" a Latin term used in ancient Greece to describe a criminal who is excluded from any rights provided to the citizens. There has not been any significant change to immigration laws in both South Africa and Botswana that would improve the situation of undocumented survival migrants.

While there are violent, intermittent xenophobic attacks in South Africa, in Botswana, undocumented immigrants are somewhat more nuanced. With migrants being referred to in a derogatory way as *makwerekwere,* or lack of access to general services. A refugee camp located on the Botswana-Zimbabwe border is infamously referred to as "*Teronko ya Zimbabwe,*" which translates to the prison for Zimbabweans. The name is derived from the number of Zimbabweans plus the poor living conditions like a prison, as there are no laws enjoining the state to provide deportees with "medical, health, or social services" (Maphosa & Ntau, 2021). Maphosa and Ntau (2021) and Moyo and Zanker (2022) detail different xenophobic slurs expressed by political personas and community leaders in South Africa, which then translate to the institutional and violent xenophobic attacks. Disappointingly, COVID-19 only exacerbated this exclusion of survival migrants.

COVID-19 and Access to ART

Although COVID-19 shed light on the flaws of the Government of Botswana system in the distribution of ART, PEPFAR had in December 2019 committed to a program that included PEPFAR Botswana Country Action Plan of Action 2020. However, its efforts were dampened by the pandemic. In its updated 2021 plan, this key aspect was included to ensure the inclusion of non-citizens in its ART programming. The policy that articulated these free clinical services to non-citizens was officially agreed to and supported by the Government of Botswana. This policy, created in line with WHO guidelines, emphasizes helping all non-citizens, despite their immigration status. With increased awareness, this would be a key intervention for survival migrants in need of such services. Even without referring to statistics, it is a necessary program that would be favorable to survival migrants.

The Pre- and Post-COVID-19 Immigration Question

One glaring question that was highlighted by COVID-19 is the effectiveness of immigration policies pertaining to economic migrants, especially in the context of South African migration. The deportation system has become "a revolving door system" (Jackson & Hoque, 2022), with the same immigrants being repeatedly deported. Further, in 2019, the South African immigration system was facing a backlog that would take 68 years for the DHA to resolve (Moyo & Zanker, 2022). Arguably, it is easier to have an ambiguous migratory system that a government can derive cheap labor from rather than legitimize the migrants and increase the burden on struggling social welfare systems. Studies have shown that including informal sectors in the economy would only benefit the GDP on a grander scale. In South Africa, the informal economy has an estimated value equivalent to 28.8 percent of its GDP (World Economics, 2022). In Botswana, the informal economy accounts for an estimated 26.7 percent of its GDP (World Economics, 2022). These informal economies are not entirely made up of survival migrant labor, but it cannot be denied that survival migrants make a significant contribution that allows the informal and formal economies to thrive.

RECOMMENDATIONS

A stagnant policy of immigration that is centered around the 1951 convention has meant that immigrants that migrate to survive do not fit within the definitions of the convention. Within the SADC region, the level of migration is so extensive that it is becoming costly to prevent the movement of survival migrants rather than to allow them to move across borders. In Botswana, a 500km fence has been constructed at the Botswana-Zimbabwe border that was allegedly aimed at avoiding animals, particularly livestock, crossing into Botswana and spreading disease (Lefko-Everett, 2004). However, this fence has been said to also prevent illegal migration into Botswana. Similarly, in South Africa, when COVID-19 began to spread, the South African government's initial reaction was to construct a 40km long fence at the Beitbridge border post. The cost of these fences could have been utilized to facilitate grants for survival migrants or added to the health care system to cater to survival migrants and avoid the continued spread of COVID-19. The Botswana Border Fence cost approximately BWP 35 million (Kopiński, 2012), while the South African Border Fence cost of R37 million to construct (BusinessTech, 2020). Exclusionary policies are outdated and are proving to be increasingly costly for both the South African and Botswana governments. Inclusionary immigration policies would allow governments to benefit economically from survival migrants by legitimizing their presence. It would also allow for holistic studies to be done to assess the real economic costs and benefits of migrants. Currently, because survival immigrants do not have legal status, the statistics are usually approximations that do not create reliable data or a full picture.

The success of exclusionary immigration policies is yet to be shown as successfully preventing entry into more developed nations. If countries in SADC continue to struggle, especially fragile states like Zimbabwe, migrants will continue to flout the laws. It can also be noted that cost of deporting survival migrants who are willing and able to earn an honest living is probably equal to, if not even more so, granting survival migrants the right to earn a living legitimately, especially when it comes to healthcare. In the Botswana context, it would cost approximately US$74 million over a decade to include migrants on free ART treatment (Carter, 2020). Although this appears like a large sum in the long run, it would minimize the continued spread of HIV and allow for the holistic implementation of the 95-95-95 targets by including all members of the community. The spread of HIV continues to be costly, and a lack of treatment also compromises one's immune system, thereby putting them at higher risk contracting COVID-19.

Regional migration policy needs to be updated to allow free movement across borders and access to welfare services if that person is employed within that country. Governments can devise bilateral agreements that would facilitate ease of migration for the ultimate benefit of all parties. For instance, Algeria, Morocco, and Tunisia have entered into agreements with destination countries wherein migrants are assured of social security and to shield them against racism and xenophobia (Ratha, Mohapatra, Ozden, Plaza, Shaw, & Shimeles, 2011). Noting the increasing costs of preventing survival migrants through fences and deportations, it is critical that the South African and Botswana governments develop bilateral agreements with their neighboring countries to remedy the gaps highlighted by the COVID-19 pandemic.

COVID-19 has highlighted the ineffectiveness of restrictive immigration policies, whereby, despite the fences that are placed and the restrictive policies, survival migrants manage to enter these countries and find work for their sustenance. The economy benefits from the labor that is paid with low wages that are not officially recorded. However, their lack of access to social protection is what negatively impacts the destination countries. For instance, in the face of COVID-19, untreated survival migrants without access to health care out of fear of exposure or otherwise would lead to the continued spread of disease.

Further, the wider impact on other economies could be a result of the exclusion of survival migrants from social protection policies. The International Monetary Fund (IMF) identifies that in 2018 alone, global remittances by migrants to their home countries reached USD 350 billion (Sayeh & Chami, 2020). The fragile states from which some of these survival migrants are coming depend on the foreign remittances sent by survival migrants. In the era of COVID-19, remittances will reduce because of restricted movement and the inability of these survival migrants to earn an income. It is recommended by Sayeh and Chami (2020) that host countries stabilize employment opportunities for migrant workers or increase their requests for donor aid from the international community. The former solution provides greater security and sustainability for survival migrants as they earn their income rather than wait for donor handouts.

CONCLUSION

The COVID-19 pandemic has placed a magnifying glass on policy and infrastructural deficits for governments worldwide, especially in the health sector. States must find themselves rethinking policies and regional integration of migration policies to allow all nations to benefit. Botswana and South Africa have the strongest economies in the SADC region. Evidence has shown that integrating migrants into their economies assists them in capacity building and the performance of menial and casual work where there is minimal competition from locals (Africa, 2018). It goes without saying that migration must be considered through a human developmental lens. There should be consideration of how survival migrants can lawfully assist the development of the state they reside in and which of their human rights need to be addressed. The era of crisis has shown how anemic the policy landscape is when it comes to migration. The ramifications of this are an undocumented, disenfranchised population with respect to health and subsistence. Contributions of legal migrants are a partial picture of immigrants who are contributors to the state despite not receiving the full benefits of paying taxes. The costs of exclusionary policies have become glaring in the era of COVID-19 and have led to the displacement of some survival immigrants and the unfortunate return of others to the situations that they were fleeing from in their home countries.

REFERENCES

Africa, M. F. *Migration Policy Framework for Africa and Plan of Action.* Addis Ababa: African Union Commission, AU Department for Social Affairs (2018).

Ankara. *Hundreds Flee from Virus Quarantine Center in Malawi.* (2020, May 28). Retrieved from AA:https://www.aa.com.tr/en/africa/hundreds-flee-from-virus-quarantine-center-in- malawi/1856275

Belin, A., Zamparutti, T., Tull, K., & Milieu, G. H. *Occupational Health and Safety Risks For The Most Vulnerable Workers.* Brussells: Directorate General For Internal Policies Policy Department A: Economic And Scientific Policy Employment And Social Affairs (2011, August).

Betts, A. *Survival Migration Failed Governance and the Crisis of Displacement.* Ithaca: Cornell University Press (2013).

Carter, M. *Excluding Migrants from HIV Programmes in Botswana is Slowing Reductions in HIV Incidence.* (2020, February 5). Retrieved from AIDS map: https://www.aidsmap.com/news/feb-2020/excluding-migrants-hiv-programmes-botswana-slowing-reductions-hiv-incidence

Centre, O. D. *How Immigrants Contribute to South Africa's Economy.* (2018, July 16). Retrieved from OECD iLibrary: http://dx.doi.org/10.1787/9789264085398-en

Center for Disease Control and Prevention. *Implementing Safety Practices for Critical Infrastructure Workers Who May Have Had Exposure to a Person with Suspected or Confirmed COVID-19.* (2020, September 11). Retrieved from https://www.cdc.gov/coronavirus/2019-ncov/community/critical-infrastructure sectors.html?CDC_AA_refVal=https%3A%2F%2Fwww.cdc.gov%2Fcoronavirus%2F2019-ncov%2Fcommunity%2Fcritical-workers%2Fimplementing-safety-practices.html

Chami, R. & Sayeh, A. *Finance and Development.* (2020, June). Retrieved from International Monetary Fund: https://www.imf.org/external/pubs/ft/fandd/2020/06/COVID19-pandemic-impact-on-remittance-flows-sayeh.htm

Dube, M. *Botswana Battles Influx Zimbabwean Illegal Immigrants.* (2019, August 14). Retrieved from Voice of America: https://www.voanews.com/africa/botswana-battles-influx-zimbabwean-illegal-immigrants

Dube, M. *Struggling Sex Workers in Botswana Get Food Aid.* (2020, May 12). Retrieved from Voice of America: https://www.voanews.com/africa/struggling-sex-workers-botswana-get-food-aid

Goitom, H. *Laws Concerning Children of Undocumented Migrants: South Africa.* (2017, September). Retrieved from Library of Congress: https://www.loc.gov/law/help/undocumented-migrants/southafrica.php

Google. (2020, September 26). *Google News.* Retrieved from google news: https://news.google.com/covid19/map?hl=enBW&mid=%2Fm%2F0166v&gl=BW&ceid=BW%3Aen

Gurumoorthi, G. *Covid 19 Botswana Government Wage Subsidy Scheme.* (2020, April 11). Retrieved from RSM Global: https://www.rsm.global/botswana/news/covid-19-botswana-government-wage-subsidy-scheme

International Labour Organisation. *Sub-Major Group 74: Other Craft and Related Trades Workers.* (2004). Retrieved from ILO: https://www.ilo.org/public/english/bureau/stat/isco/isco88/74.htm

Jackson, J. & Hoque, M. Effective Management of Deportation of Undocumented Migrants from South Africa. (2022). Retrieved from https://www.intechopen.com/chapters/80453

Kavuro, C. *South Africa Excludes Refugees and Asylum Seekers from Covid-19 Aid.* (2020, May 29). Retrieved from Mail and Guardian: https://mg.co.za/coronavirus-essentials/2020-05-29-south-africa-refugees-coronavrus-exclude-law/

Khumalo, T. *South Africa's New Immigration Laws Worry Zimbabwean Immigrants.* (2014, June 13). Retrieved from Voice of America: https://www.voanews.com/africa/s-africas-new-immigration-laws-worry-zimbabwean-immigrants

Kopiński. D. A. P. Is Botswana Creating a New Gaza Strip? An Analysis of the 'Fence Discourse' In J. T. Cristina Udelsmann Rodrigues, *Centro de Estudos Internacionais* (pp. 98–111). Lisbon: Centro de Estudos Internacionais (2012). Retrieved from https://books.openedition.org/cei/235?lang=en

Lefko-Everett, K. Botswana's Changing Migration Patterns. (2004, September 1). Retrieved from Migration Policy Institute: https://www.migrationpolicy.org/article/botswanas- changing-migration-patterns

Maphosa, F. & Ntau, C. Undocumented Migrants as *Homo Sacer*: Cases From Botswana and South Africa. *Journal of African and Asian Studies*, 56(4), (2021), 872–888. Retrieved from https://journals.sagepub.com/doi/full/10.1177/0021909620946349

Mosikare, L. *Rise in Number of Deported Zim Immigrants.* (2020, July 6). Retrieved from The Monitor: https://www.mmegi.bw/index.php?aid=86166&dir=2020/july/06

Moyo, K. & Zanker, F. No Hope for the 'Foreigners': The Conflation of Refugees and Migrants in South Africa. *Journal of Immigrant & Refugee Studies*, 20(2), (2022), 253–265. Retrieved from https://www.tandfonline.com/doi/full/10.1080/15562948.2021.2007318

Nolan, P. D. *Loss Prevention and Safety Control: Terms and Definitions.* CRC Press (2011).

PEPFAR Botswana, COP 2021Updates to Botswana's Country Operational Plan 2020 Strategic Direction Summary, May 12, 2021. Retrieved from https://www.state.gov/wp-content/uploads/2021/09/Botswana_SDS_Final-Public_Aug-11-2021.pdf

Polus, D. K. Is Botswana Creating a New Gaza Strip? An Analysis of the 'Fence Discourse'. In C. Rodrigues, *Crossing African Borders: Migration and Mobility* (pp. 98–111). Lisboa: Centro de Estudos Internacionais (2012). Retrieved from Centro de Estudos Internacionais: https://books.openedition.org/cei/235?lang=en

Ratha, D., Mohapatra, S., Ozden, C., Plaza., S., Shaw, W., & Shimeles, A. *Leveraging Migration For Africa: Remittances Skills and Investments.* Washington, DC: The International Bank for Reconstruction and Development / The World Bank (2011).

Reyburn, P. *South Africa: National Disaster Declaration – Now What?* (2020, March 26). Retrieved from ENS Africa: https://www.lexology.com/library/detail.aspx?g=820ce52a-f2ff-4f52-81e0-325a7d1650b7

Rugunanan, P. *"South Africa Belongs To All Who Live In It", COVID-19 Showed It Does Not.* (2020, July 2). Retrieved from Open Democracy: https://www.opendemocracy.net/en/pandemic- border/south-africa-belongs-to-all-who-live-in-it-covid-19-showed-it-does-not/

Runciman, C. *Gaps in South Africa's Relief Scheme Leave Some Workers with No Income.* (2020, April 22). Retrieved from The Conversation: https://theconversation.com/gaps-in-south-africas- relief-scheme-leave-some-workers-with-no-income-136403

Russ, H. *Fast Food Closures Sweep U.K., as Even Drive-Thrus Deemed Unsafe.* (2020, March 24). Retrieved December 2020, from Reuters: https://www.reuters.com/article/us-health-coronavirus-fastfood-idUSKBN21B02A

Schensema, H., Nketu, M., & York, T. *Deadline for holders of Zimbabwean Exemption Permits has been extended until 31 December 2023. (2023, June 8).* Retrieved August 2023, from Cliffe, Dekker, Hofmeyer Incoorporating Kieta Law LLP: https://www.cliffedekkerhofmeyr.com/news/publications/2023/Sectors/Immigration/immigration-law-alert-8-june-deadline-for-holders-of-zimbabwean-exemption-permits-has-been-extended-until-31-december-2023-

South African Government. *Social Grants – COVID-19.* (2020, September 5). Retrieved from www.gov.za:https://www.gov.za/covid-19/individuals-and-households/social-grants-coronavirus-covid-19

The Associate Press. *South African court rules against government over ending permits for nearly 200,000 Zimbabweans.* (2023, June). Retrieved from: https://abcnews.go.com/International/wireStory/south-african-court-rules-government-ending-permits-200000-100446362

Town, T. S. *Migrant and Refugee Access to Public Healthcare in South Africa.* (2020, September). Retrieved from The Scalabrini Centre of Cape Town: https://scalabrini.org.za/ news/migrant-and-refugee-access-to-public-healthcare-in-south-africa/

Truen, S. K. K. Updating the South Africa-SADC Remittance Channel Estimates. South Africa. (2016, December).

World Economics. *"South Africa's Informal Economy Size as a Percentage of GDP %".* https://www.worldeconomics.com/National-Statistics/Informal-Economy/South%20Africa.aspx

Chapter 7

Caught between a Rock and a Hard Place

The Impact of the COVID-19 Pandemic on Refugees in Namibia

Ananias Janet, Leonard Emma, and Chikadzi Victor

INTRODUCTION

The COVID-19 pandemic caused widespread economic, social, and political disturbances on a global scale. While many countries eased the national shutdowns that were necessitated by the crisis, the global order as we knew it is yet to be restored. The COVID-19 crisis bore witness to a redefinition of solidarity, with many countries gravitating towards national priorities as the foremost principle guiding decision-making. There are far-reaching implications of such decisions, especially for refugee communities around the globe who are caught up in pandemic crises. While nationals in all countries are indeed vulnerable, refugee communities are amongst the most vulnerable to the pandemic crisis and its attendant effects on their social and economic lives. As nations look inwards at their own citizens, one is left to wonder how life has been for refugees who are caught up in host countries in which they have become "others."

As nations looked inward as a form of national solidarity, programmatic responses to the COVID-19 pandemic necessitated that an inclusive and holistic approach be adopted, which included the very welfare of refugees. Without this, the refugee community can easily pose a serious threat to national health efforts, given that an outbreak of the disease within refugee camps and settlements may inevitably spread to local communities and beyond. The World Health Organization (2020) noted that the exclusion of refugees from national health programs and social responses has the potential, among others, to render early detection, testing, diagnosis, contact tracing, and provision of care for refugees and migrants affected by COVID-19 difficult. The crowded nature of refugee camps further exacerbates the risk of outbreaks in these population groups. Further, such outbreaks may be concealed or go unnoticed, which presents an additional threat to public health. Thus, while there has been a pronounced gravitation towards national solidarity in the face of the COVID-19 pandemic, response plans have to consider special population groups, such as refugees, given their vulnerability profile. There is an increased likelihood of the spread of the disease in camp conditions, which are commonly associated with poor infrastructure and overcrowding globally (Shrivastava and Shrivastava 2020).

Namibia is host to a small population of refugees, many of whom live in refugee settlement camps, while others are now integrated into mainstream communities. Thus far, not much is known about the experiences of refugees within Namibia during this period of the COVID-19 crisis. Against this backdrop, this chapter investigated the experiences of the refugee community in Namibia, considering the COVID-19 pandemic. As millions are gripped with fear and anxiety over what would be, it is palpable that refugee communities would be more prone to a myriad of social, economic, and psychological challenges. It was therefore necessary to explore the experiences of refugees in Namibia to better understand the unique ways in which this vulnerable population group is affected. Such an understanding is important in informing response efforts that target the socioeconomic and mental health needs of refugees in crisis situations. To this end, the chapter investigated the impact of COVID-19 on refugees in Namibia.

THE GLOBAL, AFRICAN, AND NAMIBIAN CONTEXT ON REFUGEES

As at the end of 2019, there were over 79.5 million people around the world who were displaced from their own communities due to a myriad of factors, such as war, violence, political persecution, and hunger, amongst other things (United Nations High Commission on Refugees, UNHCR 2020). Of these, it is estimated that about 26 million are refugees (UNHCR 2020). Due to a multitude of factors, Africa continues to see a marked increase in the number of people seeking refuge. Several factors, among them political violence, wars, persecution, and economic crises, account for this increase in the refugee population and other categories of immigrants. It is estimated that Sub-Saharan Africa is home to around 26 percent of the global refugee population. Most of the refugees come from countries such as South Sudan, the Central African Republic Somalia, Eritrea, Sudan, the Democratic Republic of the

Congo, and Burundi, which are largely affected by civil wars and economic instability (United Nations General Assembly 2018; UNHCR 2020). Several African countries are host to refugee populations despite the many social, economic, and political challenges these nations face (United Nations General Assembly 2018). The continued arrival of refugees in these countries is therefore an unwelcome development that adds to existing burdens they face. Most refugees in Africa reside in camps under difficult conditions (Jozaghi and Dahya 2020; Taylor et al. 2016). Many countries are reluctant to integrate refugees into mainstream society, and they favor containing them in camp settings where they are located far away from economic opportunities and have limited access to the outside world (UNHCR 2018).

Countries such as South Africa, Botswana, and Namibia are most popular destinations for refugees (Oucho 2007). The southern African region has over the years experienced modest economic growth. As such, many countries have high levels of poverty, inequality, and unemployment (UNHCR 2018). This makes the situation of refugees dire and countries facing their own domestic challenges cannot do much for 'aliens' (UNHCR 2020).

To uphold its international obligations, the Namibian government has also promulgated the Refugees (Recognition and Control) Act 2 of 1999 and Regulations (Groenewaldt 2010). The Namibia Refugees Act, under Section 3 of the Act, stipulates that a person shall be a refugee if:

(a) owing to a well-founded fear of being persecuted for reasons of race, religion, nationality, membership of a particular social group or political opinion, he or she is outside the country of his or her nationality and is unable or, owing to such fear, is unwilling to avail himself or herself of the protection of that country; or
(b) not having a nationality and being outside the country of his or her former habitual residence, he or she is unable or, owing to a well-founded fear of being persecuted for reasons of race, religion, membership of a particular social group or political opinion, is unwilling to return to it; or
(c) owing to external aggression, occupation, foreign domination or events seriously disturbing public order in either part or the whole of his or her country of origin or nationality, he or she is compelled to leave his or her place of habitual residence in order to seek refuge in another place outside his or her country of origin or nationality.

Namibia maintains its reservation to Article 26 of the 1951 Convention and consequently continues to limit the freedom of movement of refugees and asylum-seekers (Groenewaldt 2010). To that effect, Section 19 of the 1999 Namibia Refugees (Recognition and Control) Act provides that all asylum seekers and refugees may be received at the Osire refugee settlement and/or reside at any part of Namibia that is declared, gazetted, and designated as a reception or residence area, respectively. The Osire refugee settlement, a designated residential area for refugees, is located between commercial farms, some 245 kilometers from the capital, Windhoek. It is also situated about 124 kilometers from Otjiwarongo, which is the nearest town. According to the UNHCR, Namibia as of February 2015 hosted 2,603 refugees and asylum-seekers, mainly from the Democratic Republic of the Congo (2,074), followed by Burundi (266) and Rwanda (165), and the remaining from Zimbabwe and other countries (UNHCR 2015). The actual number of refugees in Namibia is, however, not known, as there is a lack of clarity on refugee statistics in the country. Consequently, the study from which this chapter culminated could not obtain current official statistics from the responsible authorities. However, the participants who were interviewed for the study estimated the number of people currently residing at Osire refugee settlement to be around 6,000.

At the Osire refugee camp, refugees need to apply for a permit from the settlement administrator before they can be allowed to leave the camp (Groenewaldt 2010; UNHCR 2015). The permits are issued on a temporary basis, and their validity is for a few days, after which the refugees have to return to the camp. If any refugee fails to return to the camp within the time limit set out on the permit, it may lead to their arrest and detention under the Immigration Control Act 7 of 1993, which is the legal instrument that stipulates regulations guiding the entry and movement of persons within the borders of Namibia. Despite the many efforts of the government of Namibia targeted at ensuring that refugees live in dignity at the Osire camp, their situation remains ominous due to limited access to land, absence of employment opportunities, and the lack of higher education opportunities for refugees (UNHCR 2015).

To date, not much has been done to provide lasting solutions for the Osire refugee population (UNHCR/WFP Joint Assessment and Evaluation Mission 2008). As of 2015, the UNHCR, which was the stakeholder involved in the administration of the Osire camp, exited Namibia and ceded control of the camp to the government (UNHCR 2015). Refugees are still receiving support through an implementing partner organization supported by the UNHCR through its South Africa office. Despite the many efforts of the implementing partner to support refugees, they remain short of essential supplies needed for survival. As such, many refugees must find ways to supplement the support they get from donors within the confines of the camp, which is difficult (UNHCR 2015).

THE COVID-19 SITUATION IN NAMIBIA

On March 17, 2020, the government of Namibia imposed a national lockdown to slow down and ultimately combat the spread of the COVID-19 virus (Government Gazette of the Republic of Namibia 2020). This, inter alia, included a prohibition relating to entry into Namibia by non-Namibians, non-permanent residence holders, persons not domiciled or ordinarily resident in Namibia, or persons who do not belong to the diplomatic community accredited to Namibia (Government Gazette of the Republic of Namibia 2020). These measures were not isolated; within the same period, neighboring countries such as Botswana, South Africa, Zimbabwe, Lesotho, and Eswatini, amongst others, did the same. As national borders were shut down, the regional supply chain of goods and services was seriously disrupted. The panic triggered by pandemic continued to take root, and national solidarity became pronounced in the measures that countries were taking to avert the pandemic reaching their borders. Movement of persons across borders was curtailed, and many countries were only allowing their nationals to come in while all other persons were banned (Government Gazette of the Republic of Namibia 2020). The halt of economic activity and movement of people did not only affect regional commerce and travel, but the movement between regions was also banned except for persons with special permits allowing them to travel.

Within Namibia, the effects of these measures on nationals have been marked. Many companies shut down or downsized operations and retrenched workers. People lost their jobs daily, while others have seen their earnings reduced. Namibians living on the margins of the mainstream economy were hardest hit in terms of the social and economic impact of the pandemic. In response, the government of Namibia announced a raft of economic and social protection measures to cushion its people (Shiimi 2020). As solidarity is defined firstly based on nationality, as evidenced in the raft of government response measures that largely focus on nationals, several population groups within the Namibian borders found themselves trapped with very limited sources of support to cope and survive the crisis. Amongst these population groups, refugees are the most vulnerable and worst affected of all. Refugees as a population group are a vulnerable category that suffers from multiple layers of disadvantage, and the COVID-19 pandemic has aggravated the already desperate situation of refugees, not only in Namibia but globally. The pandemic has had widespread social, economic, and health costs for the refugee population (Philbrick et al. 2017).

THEORETICAL FRAMEWORK

This chapter adopted the ecosystem perspective as the lens through which the phenomenon of refugees was studied. The ecosystems approach is one of the many theoretical perspectives that emerged from the general systems theory that was popularized in the 1960s (Lesser and Pope 2007). Lesser and Pope (2007, 8) further note that general systems theory is "a set of rules for analyzing how systems operate and are related to one another." In this vein, refugees and their experiences can be best studied and understood from an ecosystemic perspective, as it allows us to view them not just as individuals, but rather as individuals existing and functioning in an environment. This environment can be viewed as an ecosystem that has various subsystems within it. Thus, to holistically interrogate and document refugee experiences, one must understand the ecosystem within which they exist. The various subsystems of that ecosystem were interrogated to see how the various interactions and interrelationships of the subsystems shaped the refugee experiences. This perspective sought to understand refugees not just as persons but as persons within an environment. The environment in this instance included, but was not limited to, the camp, policies that govern refugees in Namibia, professionals that work with refugees, the economic and political environment in the country, and the health system.

STUDY METHODS

Research Paradigm and Design

A qualitative research approach was adopted in this study due to its applicability when studying human experiences from an insider perspective (Johnson and Onwuegbuzie 2004). The study explored the lived experiences of refugees, and the exploratory qualities of the qualitative research approach best suited the purposes of this study. Bryman (2008) posits that the qualitative approach is explorative in nature and makes it possible to obtain holistic and detailed participant accounts that enable researchers to answer the questions relevant to a study. Within the qualitative research paradigm, the study adopted the multiple case study design. According to (Gerring, 2007) a case study is an exhaustive and detailed study of a single or multiple cases with the purpose of obtaining a clear understanding of a particular phenomenon. Such understanding helps researchers extrapolate their findings to other similar or related cases and contexts.

Research Population, Sampling, Data Collection, and Analysis

The purposive sampling method was used to select fifteen refugees who were over the age of 18. The key criteria were that they should be living in the camp during the COVID-19 crisis and be able to communicate in English. In addition, five key informants who were professionals working with refugees were included in the sample. Semi-structured telephone interviews lasting approximately 30 minutes to an hour were conducted with the participants. The data were transcribed and then thematically analyzed.

FINDINGS AND DISCUSSION

From the empirical data gathered for this chapter, several thematic areas emerged on how refugees in Namibia have been affected by the pandemic. The discussion of the findings below is largely general information that is in the public domain and was largely conveyed via newspaper articles.

Economic Exclusion

The situation of most refugees is one of economic marginalization, and they live at the margins of the mainstream economy. Camp settlements for refugees are largely situated in remote places that have no economic opportunities. This precludes refugees from participating in productive economic initiatives. It is therefore tough for many refugees, and they find it hard to enjoy reasonable standards of living. Often, refugees struggle to meet their necessities (Hathaway and Forster 2014; Jahre et al. 2018). One of the main challenges for refugees revolves around livelihoods and survival. In most cases, the economic prospects for refugees are very limited given their disadvantaged situation and, in some cases, the constraints that are put on them by host countries. It is not uncommon for countries to treat refugees unfairly by denying them their basic rights and needs as a way of forcing them to leave while also using that as a deterrent measure for those who may want to come (Hathaway and Forster 2014). In Namibia, the Osire refugee camp, where refugees are contained, is located away from mainstream economic hubs. This could be tantamount to denying them these rights. Local integration has only been considered for Angolan refugees as part of a special dispensation since 2013 (UNHCR 2015). Within the Osire refugee settlement, the mobility of refugees is tightly controlled and monitored. Refugees must obtain permits to exit the settlement. While the settlement no doubt provides peace, security, and protection for refugees, it also comes with a myriad of limitations that could make the lives of refugees difficult. In particular, the economic participation of refugees is very limited and, in some cases, nonexistent. During interviews with participants, they noted that economic activity at the Osire refugee settlement is very limited. Windhoek and Otjiwarongo are the nearest towns where refugees can go and sell farm produce and wares as a way of supplementing their monthly food rations, which they get. Windhoek is 245 kilometers away, while Otjiwarongo is 124 kilometers away. Due to the vast distances to the nearest towns, most refugees at the Osire settlement were, in essence, already cut off from the Namibian mainstream economy even before the COVID-19 pandemic. They live on the margins of the productive economy, and their participation is largely limited to periodic vending if and when they have something to sell and are allowed to leave the camp.

As if the economic situation of refugees residing at Osire settlement was not bad enough, the COVID-19 pandemic has worsened an already dire situation by bringing economic activity for most refugees to a halt. The current prevailing lockdown has effectively cut off refugees from the already limited access they had to economic activity within and outside the refugee camp. It has reduced them to a situation where they find themselves in Namibia bodily but out of it in terms of participation. Refugees reported a dire situation in which they are struggling to cope.

Spending without Earning

One of the main ways in which refugees have been economically impacted by the COVID-19 pandemic has been the halt of business activity due to limited movement in compliance with the lockdown provisions. Before the lockdown, many refugees would go to Windhoek and Otjiwarongo to sell their wares. The money they earn while being little is very critical for their survival. The support given to refugees is limited to food rations, which need to be supplemented. The rations are only enough to provide basic survival. As such, the money earned from vending is necessary to ensure that refugees can have breakfast, clothes, toiletries, and relish, amongst other very basic necessities. With the introduction of the lockdown, movement in and out of the camp was tightly controlled and limited. In essence, this meant that refugees could no longer go and sell their wares to neighboring towns.

> We are not getting enough food sometimes I could send my wife to go and sell vegetables outside and bring something, you know, to support the family but now, right now, it has stopped completely. It has made a challenge to me and to others mostly most of the people is the same problem. (R8)
>
> It's like I am failing I am trying but because I do not have means of surviving but I know how to try me and my entire family how to try and keep ourselves safe but in terms financially I am failing that's a problem. (R7)
>
> Diet that problem last month we did not receive and when we received this July we received without sugar and you know that this portion they are giving is not enough for 30 days So it is a challenge there, there is no firewood there is not enough paraffin for cooking no charcoal outside those people who go to get charcoal they are restricted now they cannot go to get charcoal. (R9)

> Yea people who were selling for example things there they are not allowed to. Those who were selling in Soweto market they are not allowed to enter, there so these are things people are very worried about. (R4)

The selected participants clearly point to a situation where refugees must be spending in order to keep taking care of their basic needs while at the same time not being able to earn any income. Refugees have very little to no savings at all given the limited nature of their economic participation, especially when living in a camp settlement. COVID-19 has taken away the very little income supply opportunity that they had, leaving them in a desperate situation. As solidarity has globally been defined along national lines first, no income support has been extended to the refugee community to help cushion their already dire and desperate situation. According to Article 11(2) of the International Covenant on Economic, Social and Cultural Rights (ICESCR), states are obliged to ensure that they do everything possible to mitigate and relieve hunger, even in times of natural or other disasters (Groenewaldt 2010). The monthly food rations comprising of basics such as mealie meal, sugar, salt, cooking oil, and beans given to refugees are simply not enough to sustain them for a month, hence the need to supplement that basic supply. However, during the COVID-19 crisis, refugees had to make do with this very basic existence. Such a prevailing status quo has debilitating effects and implications for the welfare of refugees. While the strict lockdown at Osire is indeed a prudent health measure that is calculated to protect the refugee population from the pandemic, for refugees themselves, it is a delicate balance between health and welfare. In the current circumstances, health considerations have trumped the welfare needs of refugees, and no social security income provisions have been forthcoming from both international organizations and the Namibian government.

The failings of the Namibian government in its care for refugees are fathomable, as the nation is affected by economic constraints that make it hard to meet the needs of its citizens. Many Namibians continue to struggle to meet basic needs such as food, shelter, health, water, and sanitation (Groenewaldt 2010; Nakuta 2008). These domestic challenges might explain why Namibia may not be able to make equitable budgetary provision for refugees. Hence, Namibia's reliance on international refugee relief efforts, which in turn are funded through voluntary state contributions, resulting in no guarantee that aid will be adequate to meet refugee needs (Hathaway and Forster 2014). This leaves refugees in a dire situation in which their income savings and earning opportunities have been eroded without an alternative source or options. Very few well-established refugees are able to keep trading within the camp, albeit in a limited way. The rest have to make do with a basic and desperate existence. While the Namibian government takes measures to safeguard the health situation of refugees, thinking about the health of their economic well-being and survival will be a welcome development. A delicate balance is needed between the health situation of refugees and their welfare. The measures to save lives over livelihoods will, at some point, affect the very lives we seek to save. The longer the lockdown continues, the more desperate the situation for refugees will become.

Disrupted Supply Chain and Rising Costs

Another key factor that has led to worsening economic exclusion of refugees has been the disruption of transportation of goods due to the closure of borders. Several refugees rely on the regional trade networks. During the interviews with refugees and key informants, it was established that many refugees order wares from neighboring countries such as South Africa, Zambia, Botswana, and Angola, amongst others. However, due to border closures, most transportation has been limited to goods considered to be essential. This has in essence totally disrupted the supply chain, thereby affecting the economic activity of refugees and taking away the only means through which they earn income to sustain their families. Closely linked to the disruption of the supply chain has been the continued rise in prices of basic necessities at Osire refugee settlement. The very limited supplies that are reaching the camp are being sold at a premium. Transport costs have gone up, and this in turn affects pricing. On the other hand, limited movement of transport within Namibia also means that the supply of goods is affected, leading to artificial shortages that have a knock-on effect on the prices of goods and services. Beyond the normal cost drivers, people, by nature, will always take advantage of crisis situations in order to profit. In this regard, the situation at the Osire refugee settlement makes it easy for "privileged persons" who have goods in stock to adopt predatory pricing models.

> Yea for the time being the only complaint people are having is that they cannot go out as often as they wish because they are restricted they cannot go every day the way they were doing and for them apart from what is distributed as food they need also food from outside mostly food from Windhoek so if it's not entering here then everything locally will be more expensive than usual yea so that is something people are complaining about. (K 4)
>
> People have days for shopping. Normally it used to be every day but now because of COVID it's reduced. You can only go Monday, if there is a trip, or Wednesday and Friday. Many people have small businesses in the camp and they don't get enough for their shop. Sometimes when you go there to buy something there is nothing that they have at that time. And also most of

them sell stuff to us the professionals, so sometimes because they cannot go to Windhoek and only seven people can fit in a van so there is a big restriction on transport. (K1)

There are restrictions in order to protect our lives [you cannot] get what you were supposed to get from town by now it is very hard, it is very hard, it is very hard for sure. (R1)

The accounts above from participants clearly show how the economic activities of refugees have been severely impacted by the COVID-19 pandemic. It is ironic that at a time when most refugees are finding themselves unable to earn money, the very little money they have is also eroded quickly due to rising costs of goods and services. This is clearly a population group suffering from multiple layers of disadvantage. Their situation is very different from that of Namibian nationals and other immigrant categories, who are at least able to still roam free, although under limited circumstances. Nationals and other immigrants can at least trade, and they also have options in terms of where they want to buy their goods. Such a luxury is a distant reality for the refugee population. In these times of global and national crisis, clearly refugees are fast becoming the "forgotten other" whose welfare needs and considerations come last.

With regards to the disruption of the supply chain and the rising costs of goods, there is a need for government intervention on humanitarian grounds to put in place measures that will cushion refugees. There is a need to ensure that a steady supply of basic necessities is facilitated, and predatory pricing, especially of basic goods, should be discouraged through either reasonable policing or providing alternative emergence retail outlets at the Osire refugee settlement. This would ensure that unnecessary travel to Windhoek and Otjiwarongo is further limited while at the same time giving relief to a vulnerable population that finds itself having to re-experience traumatic circumstances like the situations that led to them fleeing their own countries in the first place. We may all be affected by COVID-19, but economic inequality worsens its impact on others. In this regard, refugees are most affected.

COVID-19 and the Mental Health of Refugees

Refugees can be characterized as a population in crisis. They leave their home countries due to varied circumstances. Thus, in many ways, many people who seek refuge in other countries are traumatized and fearful (Mattar and Piwowarczyk 2020, S228–S229). While the peaceful situation in the receiving countries is a welcome break from war situations and other forms of abuse, the disruption of life caused by fleeing is something that is not easily shaken off and is therefore a source of stress and possible trauma. To this end, refugees have mental health needs perhaps much greater than any other population group. Before the COVID-19 pandemic, the refugee situation at Osire was characterized by refugees as fair and acceptable compared to where they ran away from, although it was still a difficult way of surviving. As already alluded to, refugees at Osire were largely cut off from the mainstream Namibian economy and had very limited means of survival outside of the food rations they received monthly (Pinehas, Van Wyk, and Leech 2016, 140). This makes their situation desperate, and the current pandemic multiplies the burden. This has debilitating effects on the mental health of refugees. The economic impact and social costs of the pandemic are weighing very heavily and disproportionally on the refugee population. It is simply adding to and compounding their already stressful existence. The main sources of stress for refugees due to COVID-19 restrictions are, but not limited to, limited movement, reduced economic activity, eroded livelihoods, fear and anxiety, and rising costs of living amongst other things.

On the other hand, just before the global lockdown was imposed, a number of refugees were already in their final stages of relocation to several overseas destinations. Many were awaiting their departure dates, having already sold their few belongings. Now they are having to nurse dashed hopes and uncertainty and, at the same time, deal with the fact that they have to start afresh to reconstruct their livelihoods at the camp. This is clearly an unbearable situation, which no doubt affects the mental health of refugees. Such has been the impact of the COVID-19 pandemic.

> First of all us refugees you are a traumatized person so you are already having problems and now with those problems you find yourself in this pandemic then fear is there. (R11)
>
> Yea the stress of course is there and fear people are really fearing most of them if you hear them praying it is let COVID not reach Osire we are already having a lot of problems here not talk of this death and other catastrophes fear is there in and people are stressed. (R7)
>
> The way I see things is people are very worried. Some of them they were thinking going abroad is where they will find solution to their life to their future but abroad is also a problem because they don't also want to receive people coming from outside because of the same pandemic so this one is making them to become very worried and we are having people who were supposed to travel to go to America for resettlement but now it is blocked they can no more go there we don't know up to when so worry is there and also people cannot find work they cannot work so its worrying them. Some are trying to go outside to work but if you are outside there then to get work is difficult we are hearing from outside that since COVID started refugees are not treated the way they were treated before this was from people who are outside especially in Windhoek. (R10)

It is clear from the selected participants' accounts above that the mental health of refugees is under a serious strain. Worryingly, COVID-19 has no cure, and a healthy immune system is argued to be the best chance of survival, yet stress weakens the immune system and may reduce the survival chances of some refugees should the virus spread in the camp (Liang, Zhu, and Fang 2020, 867–877). While many refugees have had to cope with what could be deemed difficult and traumatic situations, the reality is that COVID-19 may prove to be an even worse experience. Globally, thousands of people continue to die on a daily basis (Roy and Ghosh 2020, 2). What does this mean for refugees at Osire? It's a refugee camp with very limited control measures, and should the virus spread in the camp, it could easily lead to a catastrophe. Social distancing and isolation within a refugee camp situation are proving to be a challenge. For those people who are literate and have a better grasp of what is at stake, the worry and fear are real. This is creating a "siege" situation in which refugees find themselves vulnerable and defenseless. In a crisis like COVID-19, it is palpable for refugees to feel more anxious and under siege due to fear and uncertainty. Information gaps can also increase feelings of vulnerability and helplessness, leading to stress. Triantafyllou et al. (2018, 232) note that immigration is often a very stressful event for young people and their families, both during the process of immigration and in the aftermath of the relocation and settling period. During this time, refugees are saddled with the challenge of having to adapt to a new and often hostile environment that is very different from the socioeconomic and cultural environment they would have been used to. In this regard, the already delicate situation of refugees is further worsened by the COVID-19 crisis.

Compromised Access to Health Services and Protective Gear

In terms of the WHO guidelines on the management of the COVID-19 pandemic, equitable access to health services and nondiscrimination are two of the key measures that need to be ensured for all people (World Health Organization 2020, 2). After all, the health of all classes and persons in society is tied to each other. It is therefore in the interest of all that all persons should be adequately cared for. In Namibia, the government and civil society organizations are working to ensure that the welfare of refugees with regard to their health is adequately catered for (Pinehas 2014). Participants noted that since the beginning of the outbreak, a lot of efforts have been put into ensuring that the health needs of refugees were adequately met. However, it is not enough. Many refugees have no source of income to be able to afford protective items such as masks and sanitizers. On the other hand, limited movement of persons in and out of the camp means that many sick refugees who may have wanted to access health services that cannot be provided for at the camp clinic may not be able or would be reluctant to do so. In the past, Osire had a health center with a full-time medical doctor on site and possibility of inpatient admissions. However, due to the reduced population of refugees, the health center was downgraded to a clinic, and all severe cases and hospital admissions are referred to Otjiwarongo. In many ways, being far away from well-equipped medical facilities puts refugees at a disadvantage compared to other persons in the country who can freely move around.

> The challenge is the medicine. Here we do not have a hospital, we have a clinic. In our clinic we have only multivitamin and panado we don't have all the medicine that can satisfy the sick people when they get sick with that Corona. . . ." The [clinic] had small stock of masks which were given to the sick people who were there the day the masks came. It is not everybody who has a mask here at Osire. The day when corona cases are reported, I don't think our clinic will be able to take care of the cases. (R3)
>
> Due to the shortage, tailors produce masks for sale but it seems to be unaffordable for most refugees and thus the call for free distribution through the health centre "It would be much better to get it from the hospital because you know refugees here, not everybody has the capacity to get that N$10 that it is needed. . . . Today we will have our food distribution point, imagine people are coming, people are a lot, some are coming without masks, and you don't know the temperatures of everyone. (R1)
>
> Yes, for health as well we have an only clinic and you know that we are more than 3000/4000 here at the camp. So when you get sick or you cannot be transferred to Otjiwarongo or Windhoek because of this Covid 19 quarantine. So its affection also for our health in that way. And the clinic which we are having there is no medicine at all. (R8)

It is clear from the participants' accounts above that some refugees could not afford to procure masks. While efforts from the authorities to distribute masks should be acknowledged, it is still concerning that there are refugees who go around the camp without protective masks due to insufficient supply of masks. This puts them at risk, and they also endanger the lives of others. A recent study by (Islam and Yunus 2020) found that the wearing of facemasks and regular handwashing were secondary considerations for many refugees in Bangladesh. This was not only due to a lack of supply but also to ignorance and a failure to take the threat of the pandemic seriously. On the other hand, the failure to afford facemasks puts into perspective the desperate economic situation that some refugees find themselves in. Apart from masks, other essentials such as hand sanitizers are also not accessible to many refugees. While soap has been provided, one cannot always carry soap around. A lack of such protective essentials increases the chances of transmission of the COVID-19 virus. Lack of access to sanitizers is also common amongst many Namibian nationals throughout the country. As noted by Cloete (2016), factors such as affordability continue to hinder some essential hygiene practices. However, the difference is that a camp situation may require more protective measures given that it is a vulnerable setting in which the spread of the COVID-19 virus could be difficult to contain. Similarly, the lack of a well-equipped hospital facility for a camp setting that participants noted is accommodating over 6,000 people is rather worrying. If it happens that Otjiwarongo and Windhoek health care centers get overwhelmed, refugees could easily find themselves in a situation where accessing health care could be a challenge, leading to fatalities in the Osire community. On the other hand, sick people may be reluctant to seek medical attention for conditions that might need referrals due to fear of having to be admitted far away from family and acquaintances.

The prevailing health care situation at Osire is not necessarily dire; however, in this era of COVID-19, a lot of things could go wrong under current health care arrangements. This situation is not uncommon in many places globally. Scholars such as (Júnior et al. 2020) note that healthcare service provision in many humanitarian settings is normally poor and characterized by a shortage of medicines and a lack of adequately equipped facilities. As such, COVID-19 could lead to disastrous consequences in refugee camps (Hopman, Allegranzi, and Mehtar 2020, 1550). Similar concerns are put forward by (Bhagat et al. 2020, 711). They argue that developing countries have poorly equipped health care facilities, which, if overwhelmed, will affect refugees the most given national solidarity considerations.

While the health infrastructure at Osire may be deemed to be deficient, this is not uncommon in many refugee camps globally. Scholars such as Philbrick et al. (2017, 656) posit that millions of migrants are largely excluded from mainstream health service delivery initiatives in their host country and often have to rely on services that are offered by organizations operating within the voluntary sector. With ever-dwindling philanthropic dollars, resources are minimal, which means that migrant populations and refugees in particular often have to survive under conditions of deprivation and lack. Such conditions, we note, are especially dangerous and make refugees more susceptible to being infected with the coronavirus. Raju and Ayeb-Karlsson (2020, 515) note that refugee camps are usually constructed as a temporary measure, yet many of such temporary camps have now been in existence for many decades. Should the corona virus spread in such poor camp conditions, it could easily turn into a catastrophe given that the housing conditions in camp sites make it easier for infectious diseases to spread faster.

Health Risks to Persons with Underlying Health Conditions

Apart from the health concerns of refugees as a homogeneous population group, there are subcategories of persons who can be classified as vulnerable groups within a vulnerable population. These include people with underlying conditions such as diabetes, people living with HIV, and disabled people. These people have some special dietary requirements and care considerations that they may need. In a crisis like the current one, such vulnerable population groups can easily have their needs forgotten or not prioritized.

> There are people that are diabetic, sometimes they are required to eat less salty food and oily food. In order for them to go to town they have to get a letter to travel or they would not be allowed to travel at all. And if you not allowed you stay and you just have to eat what is available. Osire does not have its own shops like shopping centres. This also applies for pregnant women. There is not enough clothing here in the camp. Actually, there is none. Whatever we get is from outside. Kids were not properly dressed during winter time and these people they also don't have money to provide for themselves. (K1)
>
> Some people here have HIV and they need a good diet some of those things they buy in Windhoek now it is not easy for them to go. They are failing to sell anything to get money so it is hard for them. (R9)

The verbatim quotes above clearly speak to the need for mainstreaming vulnerabilities even in situations where one is dealing with an already vulnerable population group. The movement restrictions and lack of economic activity are no doubt having adverse effects on people with special conditions (Guadagno 2020, 4–5). They cannot get their regular supply of food provisions that address their unique needs. In cases where these provisions may be found, the cost may be prohibitive, especially given that economic activity has been halted for many refugees and they no longer have a way to earn income. Thus, programming in humanitarian emergencies has to be sensitive to special population groups such as children, the elderly, the sick, and the disabled, amongst other categories. These people are amongst the silent victims, whose voices will hardly be heard. There is a need for organizations dealing with refugees and the government of Namibia to make special considerations for all people with special needs and not deal with refugees as a homogenous group during this current crisis.

IMPLICATIONS FOR POLICY AND PRACTICE

The results of this study have several implications, both for policy and practice. A discussion of these implications is informed by the ecosystems perspective, which is the theoretical framework that informed the study.

At a policy level, the Namibian stance on hosting refugees in a camp setting needs review. Refugee camps were initiated decades ago and were designed as a short-term solution to provide for the care of refugees, while lasting solutions are being explored. Yet, refugee camps have become permanent establishments in several countries as refugees continue to proliferate (UNHCR 2016), as is the case in Namibia. While it is within the rights of any country to have the self-determination to choose its options for refugees, the COVID-19 pandemic is once again showing the precariousness of settling refugees in camp-like situations. Even though safety and protection from harm may be ensured, life and living consist of much more than a bare existence, which is what the majority of refugees living in camp conditions are exposed to. In many ways, it is a tacit denial of their being.

On the other hand, it is important that countries within SADC come up with more durable solutions to the problem of refugees. A more durable solution requires that the root causes leading to people fleeing from their own countries be tackled. Refugee camps only deal with the symptoms of the problem, and it is akin to providing first aid without administering the treatment that will lead to full recovery. The political economy of the SADC region needs a rethink. The camaraderie posture that SADC and the African Union (AU) have adopted over the years has led to a failure to confront and tackle the socioeconomic and political instability in African countries, which has led to the refugee crisis situation (Lalbahadur 2017, 4). Drawing from the ecosystems perspective, Africa can be viewed as a system. It has subsystems (countries). Any problem within a subsystem (country) will affect the entire ecosystem (continent). To this end, SADC and AU need to actively confront and tackle regional and continental problems in any country that may lead to the disruption of people, thereby causing a migration crisis. Political leaders should not be allowed to claim sovereignty while misgoverning their countries because the problems they cause will ultimately lead to crises and problems for other countries. Good governance is central to the peace and security of nations. It has to be actively pursued by all African countries, and those that fail should be helped to comply. This, in our view, will provide a lasting solution to the problem of refugees and asylum seekers. All other efforts are minimal in impact and not helpful in the long run.

At a practice level, the mental health services for refugees are being provided for by social workers at the Osire refugee settlement. It is clear that the COVID-19 pandemic has severely and negatively affected the mental health of many refugees. Therapeutic help under such circumstances is very little help if it is not accompanied by tangible material support. Tangible measures need to be put in place to ease the mental burdens caused by the pandemic on refugees. The stressors are largely material in nature, and social work interventions that holistically address such situations are needed. This means that provision of goods and services that ease the burden ought to be prioritized over any other superficial forms of therapeutic support that fail to address the root causes of possible stress and trauma amongst refugees.

POST-COVID-19 IMPLICATIONS

COVID-19 is still a current and ongoing threat to the refugee and global population. Beyond the policy and practice implications that have been discussed in the section above, we further propose the following recommendations:

The phenomenon of refugees remains a global crisis, and international aid relief received by host countries remains inadequate to provide for the socioeconomic needs of refugees. Hence, international support for aid organizations needs to be increased drastically. In order to adequately respond to global pandemics in the future, such as COVID-19, preventative measures need to be put in place to deal with the harsh living conditions that are still prevalent in refugee camps. In the aftermath of COVID-19, mental health challenges that existed before the pandemic are still present; hence, innovative mental health interventions could be considered to mitigate the distress experienced by refugees as a vulnerable population. Further research needs to be carried out on a larger scale to further understand the complex circumstances of refugees in other continental or global settings, especially during added crisis situations such as pandemics.

On the other hand, there is a need for countries to rethink the issue of refugee camps after the COVID-19 pandemic. Refugee camps have proven to be inhumane spaces of stay, and they deprive refugees of dignity and the ability to have a livelihood. Most refugee camps tend to be located away from major towns, far away from economic opportunities that would give them a livelihood. To this end, countries need to pursue the integration of refugees into local populations as their main policy position in order to avoid the human suffering caused by the constrained space of refugee camps.

Lastly, the refugee crisis is largely exacerbated by political and economic instability in many African countries. There is therefore a need for the African Union to ensure that they intervene to restore order and proper functioning in countries where most refugees are emanating from. Once political regimes know that they can be removed through the African Union, it will force them to govern responsibly and to respond adequately to the concerns of their people, thereby lessening the burden of refugees. There also needs to be a mechanism that forces countries to pay for the upkeep of their citizens when they seek refuge in other countries. This will also indirectly contribute to improved and responsive governance by many governments as they seek to ensure that their own people stay in their own countries to avoid the burden of paying.

CONCLUSION

The aim of this chapter was to discuss the impact of the COVID-19 pandemic on the welfare of refugees in Namibia. It is clear from the foregoing discussion that refugees find themselves in a very difficult situation owing to the restrictions that have been put in place to prevent the coronavirus from spreading. The current measures to safeguard the health of refugees are indeed a welcome development. Sadly, these very same measures are compromising the already compromised economic and social wellbeing of refugees. Before the pandemic, refugees at Osire settlement were already marginalized and isolated from economic opportunities. Now that the pandemic is worsening an already dire situation, not much is being done to cushion refugees apart from providing basic food supplies. Refugees are arguably the most vulnerable population group. To this end, efforts need to be put in place to cushion them from the impact of lockdown restrictions. It is never by choice that one finds themselves a refugee. They too have rights; they too need care, and effort should be made to safeguard their dignity and worth as persons.

REFERENCES

Bhagat, Ram B., Reshmi, R. S., Sahoo, Harihar, Roy, K. Archana, and Govil, Dipti. The COVID-19, migration and livelihood in India: Challenges and policy issues. *Migration Letters* 17, no. 5: 705–718. (2020). https://doi.org/10.33182/ml.v17i5.1048

Bryman, Alan. *Social Research Methods*. New York: Oxford University Press, 2008.

Cloete, L. Many Namibians lack proper sanitation. *The Namibian*, October 18, 2016. https://www.namibian.com.na/157017/archive-read/Many-Namibians-lack-proper-sanitation

Gerring, John. *Case Study Research: Principles and Practises*. New York: Cambridge University Press, 2007.

Government Gazette of the Republic of Namibia. *No 7159 – State of Emergency – COVID-19 Regulations: Namibian Constitution*. March 28, 2020. https://gazettes.africa/gazettes/na-government-gazette-dated-2020-03-28-no-7159

Groenewaldt, Angelique L. A critical assessment of Namibian refugee law in light of global and regional trends of refugee migration. MA thesis, University of Namibia, 2010. https://repository.unam.edu.na/bitstream/handle/11070/504/groenewaldt2010.pdf?sequence=1

Guadagno, Lorenzo. *Migrants and the Covid-19 Pandemic: An Initial Analysis*. 2020. https://publications.iom.int/system/files/pdf/mrs-60.pdf

Hathaway, James C., and Michelle, Foster. *The Law of Refugee Status*. Cambridge: Cambridge University Press, 2014. https://assets.cambridge.org/9781107012516_frontmatter.pdf (cambridge.org)

Hopman, Joost, Allegranzi, Benedetta, and Mehtar, Shaheen. Managing COVID-19 in low- and middle-income countries. *JAMA* (2020): n. page.

Islam, Mohammad M., and Yunus, Md Y. Rohingya refugees at high risk of Covid-19 in Bangladesh. *The Lancet Global Health* 8, no. 8 (2020): e993–e994. https://doi.org/10.1016/S2214-109X(20)30282-5

Ivakhnyuk, Irina V. Coronavirus pandemic challenges migrants worldwide and in Russia. *Population and Economics* 4, no. 2 (2020): 49–55. https://doi.org/10.3897/popecon.4.e53201

Jahre, Marianne, Kembro, Joakim, Adjahossou, Anicet, and Altay, Nezih. Approaches to the design of refugee camps: An empirical study in Kenya, Ethiopia, Greece, and Turkey. *Journal of Humanitarian Logistics and Supply Chain Management* 8, no. 3 (2018): 323–345. https://doi.org/10.1108/JHLSCM-07-2017-0034

Johnson, R. Burke, and Onwuegbuzie, Anthony J. Mixed methods research: A research paradigm whose time has come. *Educational Researcher* 33, no. 7 (2004): 14–26. https://doi.org/10.3102/0013189X033007014

Jozaghi, Ehzan, and Dahya, Azim. Refugees, asylum seekers and COVID-19: Canada needs to do more to protect at-risk refugees during the current pandemic. *Canadian Journal of Public Health* 111 (2020): 413–414. https://doi.org/10.17269/s41997-020-00357-8

Júnior, Jucier G., de Sales, Jair P., Moreira, Marcial M., Pinheiro, Woneska R., Lima, Carlos K. T., and Neto, Modesto L. R. A crisis within the crisis: The mental health situation of refugees in the world during the 2019 coronavirus (2019-nCoV) outbreak. *Psychiatry Research* 288: 113000. https://doi.org/10.1016/j.psychres.2020.113000

Lalbahadur, Aditi. *Improving SADC Responses to Bring Peace to the DRC*. October 3, 2017. https://media.africaportal.org/documents/saia_spb_166_L_albahadur_20171101.pdf

Lesser, Joan G., and Pope, Donna S. *Human Behaviour and the Social Environment: Theory and Practice*. New York: Pearson Education, 2007.

Liang, Xiao, Zhu, Yuncheng, and Fang, Yiru. COVID-19 and post-traumatic stress disorder: A vicious circle involving immunosuppression. *CNS Neuroscience & Therapeutics* 26, no. 8 (2020): 876–878. https://doi.org/10.1111/cns.13431

Mattar, Sandra, and Piwowarczyk, Linda A. COVID-19 and U.S.-based refugee populations: Commentary. *Psychological Trauma: Theory, Research, Practice, and Policy* 12, no. S1 (2020): S228–S229. http://dx.doi.org/10.1037/tra0000602

Nakuta, John. *The Justifiability of Social, Economic and Cultural Rights in Namibia and the Role of Non-Governmental Organisations*, 2008. https://www.kas.de/upload/auslandshomepages/namibia/HumanRights/nakuta.pdf

Oucho, John O. *Migration in Southern Africa: Migration Management Initiatives for SADC Member States*, 2007. https://issafrica.org/01-dec-07-iss-paper-157-migration-in-southern-africa.-migration-management-initiatives-for-sadc-member-states-john-o-oucho

Philbrick, Ann M., Wicks, Cherilyn M., Harris, Ila M., Shaft, Grant M., and Van Vooren, James S. Make refugee health care great [again]. *American Journal of Public Health* 107 (2017): 656–658. http://dx.doi.org/10.2105/AJPH.2017.303740

Pinehas, Lucia N. *Health Care Needs of Displaced Women Living in Osire Refugee Camp in Namibia*. PhD diss., University of Pretoria, 2014. https://www.mcours.net/eng/khadengrapp295.pdf

Pinehas, Lucia N., Van Wyk, Neltjie C., and Leech, Ronell. Healthcare needs of displaced women: Osire refugee camp, Namibia. *International Nursing Review* 63, no. 1 (2016): 139–147. https://doi.org/10.1111/inr.12241

Raju Emmanuel, and Sonja, Ayeb-Karlsson. Covid-19: How do you self-isolate in a refugee camp? *International Journal of Public Health* 65 (2020): 515–517.

Roy, Satyaki, and Ghosh, Preetam. Factors affecting COVID-19 infected and death rates inform lockdown-related policymaking. *Plos One* 15, no. 10 (2020). https://doi.org/10.1371/journal.pone.0241165

Shiimi, Iipumbu. *Media Statement – Economic Stimulus and Relief Package: Impact of COVID-19 on the Economy and Households*, April 1, 2020. https://mof.gov.na/documents/35641/36580/Phase+1+VF+Stimulus+and+Relief+Package%2C+Republic+of+Namibia.pdf/9a2314de-4b39-00a1-b8bd-4ffcfe1f20d3

Shrivastava, Saurabh R., and Shrivastava, Prateek S. Effective containment of the COVID-19 pandemic among migrants and refugee: World health organization. *Turkish Journal of Family Medicine and Primary Care* 14, no. 2 (2020): 163–165. https://dergipark.org.tr/tr/download/article-file/1094055

Taylor, J. Edward, Filipski, Matheusz J., Alloush, Mohamad, Gupta, Anubhab, Valdes, Ruben I. R., and Gonzalez-Estrada, Ernesto. Economic impact of refugees. *PNAS* 113, no. 27 (2016): 7449–7453. https://doi.org/10.1073/pnas.1604566113

Triantafyllou, Kalliopi, Othiti, I., Xylouris, George, Moulla, V., Ntre, Vasiliki, Kovani, Panagiota, Gertsou, I., and Anagnostopoulos, Dimitris. (2018). Mental health and psychosocial factors in young refugees, immigrants an Greeks: A retrospective study. *Psychiatriki* 29: 231–239. Available at https://doi.org/10.22365/jpsych.2018.293.231

UNHCR/WFP Joint Assessment and Evaluation Mission, Osire Refugee Camp, Namibia, February 29, 2008. https://reliefweb.int/report/angola/unhcrwfp-joint-assessment-and-evaluation-mission-osire-refugee-camp-namibia.

United Nations General Assembly. *Assistance to Refugees, Returnees and Displaced Persons in Africa: Report of the Secretary-General*, August 21, 2018. https://reliefweb.int/sites/reliefweb.int/files/resources/A_74_322_E.pdf

United Nations High Commissioner for Refugees. *Figures at a Glance*, June 16, 2022. https://www.unhcr.org/figures-at-a-glance.html

United Nations High Commissioner for Refugees. *Global Focus: 2017 End Year Report*, July 25, 2018. https://reporting.unhcr.org/sites/default/files/pdfsummaries/GR2017-SouthernAfrica-eng.pdf.

United Nations High Commissioner for Refugees. *Global Report 2016*. https://reporting.unhcr.org/sites/default/files/gr2016/pdf/Book_GR_2016_ENGLISH_complete.pdf

United Nations High Commissioner for Refugees. *UNHCR Submission on Namibia: UPR 24th Session*, June 2015. https://www.refworld.org/docid/5a12da042.html

World Health Organisation. *Preparedness, Prevention and Control of Coronavirus Disease (COVID-19) for Refugees and Migrants in Non-Camp Settings*, April 17, 2020. https://www.who.int/publications/i/item/preparedness-prevention-and-control-of-coronavirus-disease-(covid-19)-for-refugees-and-migrants-in-non-camp-settings

Chapter 8

Deep-Rooted Poverty and Inequalities in Namibia

COVID-19 Revelations

Awarab Marvin

INTRODUCTION

Poverty and inequality are the scars left by the events of the pre-colonial past in most African countries. Namibian history paints a picture about the past where those that colonized African countries were wealthy, while the masses being colonized lived in severe poverty. The colonizers dictated the victims of colonialism. The atrocities to which Africans were subjected to range from slavery, forced labor, mass killings, poverty, and degrading treatment. Namibia was not spared from experiencing the negative effects and painful events of colonialism. The Herero and Nama genocides evidence the atrocities on the part of Namibia. Namibia firstly being colonized by Germany and later taken over by South Africa, fought hard to achieve its independence. The formation of the constituent assembly led to the adoption of the Constitution. On March 21, 1990, following free and fair democratic elections, Namibia gained independence.

Independence in Namibia came with the adoption of the supreme constitution (Article 1 (6)). The Namibian people, who previously were denied fundamental rights, are now bestowed with rights and freedoms guaranteed under the Bill of Rights of the Constitution. The fact that the Constitution of Namibia has a chapter dedicated to rights and freedoms of Namibia shows the seriousness with which the drafters of the Namibian Constitution sought to afford Namibians with a dignified life where each person would exercise his or her rights and enjoy freedoms in a democratic country. Rights such as the right to life, right to liberty, respect for human dignity, and equality are indicators that the forerunners of independence sought to put an end to the autocratic and dictatorship way of doing things. Fundamental freedoms such as the right to business or occupation aim to uplift the living conditions of those hit hardest by colonialism.

LEGISLATIVE REFORMS TO ADDRESS POVERTY

Article 23(2) of the Namibia Constitution, which deals with affirmative action, empowers the legislative branch of government to enact laws aimed achieving affirmative action in Namibia. The post-independent government has thus enacted various laws and adopted various policies with the aim of addressing the political, social and economic ills of the past. The constitution being the primary source from which all legislation derives their legitimacy, provides key guiding principles to assist with legislative reforms guaranteeing reduction of inequality. Thus, Article 16 of the Constitution deals with the aspects of aquiring and disposing property; Article 23 which seeks to undo the effects of apartheid and guarantee affirmative action; Article 95 advocates for the promotion of the welfare of the people; Article 98 which provides guidelines on the principles of economic order in Namibia Article and Article 100 vest the ownership of all land, water and natural resources in the the state, if not otherwise lawfully owned. These are the key Constitutional provisions that can be used as a roadmap in crafting legislation towards economic development in Namibia.

NEW EQUITABLE ECONOMIC EMPOWERMENT FRAMEWORK

In responding to the constitutional call of ensuring affirmative action, the Namibian law-marking body approved the New Equitable Economic Empowerment Framework (NEEEF). NEEEF's aim is to advance the lives of people within Namibia who have been socially, economically, and educationally disadvantaged by the past discriminatory laws or practices. In other words, the idea is to redress the social and economic imbalances that were asserted by those in power on the poor during colonial times. The NEEEF, therefore, embodies a group of policies that are much needed to achieve greater equity in society. This is very important because no society can achieve social and economic equality without laws dealing with equity. Although this is a much-needed reform in Namibia, to achieve this well-defined funding mechanisms are required, and thus participation of all stakeholders within the public and private sectors is crucial.

Once fully enforced and implemented, the NEEEF will promote transformation in business through six empowerment pillars: Ownership; Management

Control and Employment Equity; Human Resources and Skills Development; Entrepreneurship Development and Marketing; Corporate Social Responsibilities and Value Addition; and Technology and Innovation. The ultimate aim for NEEEF is therefore to create vehicles for empowerment and remove barriers to socioeconomic advancement in order to enable previously disadvantaged persons to access productive assets and opportunities for empowerment. There are a host of other legislative and policy imperatives that have been enacted in Namibia to redress the inequalities created by the apartheid government.

Namibia, having enacted laws and policies, still has a majority of people living in extreme poverty. Many Namibians are exposed to deplorable conditions on a daily basis. Some do not even have proper housing and thus live in shacks. Others do not have basic water and ablution facilities. A clear example was found in Walvis Bay, which can be termed as a "twaloloka disaster" where approximately 100 households were left homeless. Having 100 households living in shacks in a town of 67 000 people is concerning, given that these are not the only people living in shacks, as there are also other locations within Walvis Bay with people living in shacks. The majority of the people who are located in the Okahandja Park location in Windhoek and the DRC location in Swakopmund, for example, are victims of poverty. COVID-19 has not initiated poverty and consequences attached thereto but has simply magnified the difficulties people face daily because of poverty.

AFFIRMATIVE ACTION (EMPLOYMENT) ACT, 1998 (ACT 29 OF 1998)

The Affirmative Action Act was enacted in response to Article 23 of the constitutional, which necessitates the enactment of legislation seeking to redress the inequalities of the past. The purpose of this Act is to redress the conditions and sufferings of persons in the employment context, where such persons have been identified to form part of designated groups of persons. This is to be done through appropriate affirmative action. A critical analysis of whether this Act has achieved its mandate falls outside the scope of this chapter. It is, however, needless to state that Namibia has adhered laws to combat inequalities. The implementation of such laws, however, needs serious rethinking.

OUTBREAK AND EFFECTS OF THE PANDEMIC

The novel coronavirus disease known as COVID-19 first broke out in Wuhan City of China in the late 2019. It is a viral infection caused by severe acute respiratory syndrome, which can be transmitted from one person to the next quickly and at a very high rate with devastating effects (Adefisoye & Adefisoye, 2020, pp. 15–31). The COVID-19 pandemic continues to adversely affect the already weak and fragile world economy, as it has pulled the world economy into a recession with the potential of deep consequences of unemployment. In March 2020, the Namibian president, like the heads of state of most other countries, and as empowered by Article 26(1) of the Constitution declared as State of Emergency and put in place necessary measures to contain the spread of the disease. Measures mostly included quarantines, travel restrictions, and lockdowns of cities with the rapid spread of the pandemic, and this resulted in a significant reduction in demand and supply (WHO, 2020).

In the case of *Namibian Employers' Federation v President of the Republic of Namibia* (HC-MD-CIV-MOT-GEN-2020/00136) [2020] NAHCMD 248 (23 June 2020), the High Court held that Article 26 of the Constitution may serve, where appropriate, to suspend the exercise and enjoyment of some fundamental rights prescribed by the Constitution. One wonders whether there is a limit in scope to the powers of the president in such an instance and whether there is any balancing act applied in the application of Article 26. In Namibia, the capital city and the harbor towns of Walvis and Swakopmund have been under lookdowns. Most economic activities of sale and purchase of goods as well as imports and exports, mostly take place at Walvis Bay and Windhoek. Placing these towns under lockdown had severe consequences for the economy of the country and the livelihoods of people. The government redirected funds and resources to respond quickly to the rapid spread of the pandemic. Funds that would otherwise have been used for other economic activities have now continuously been used for preventing the spread of the pandemic.

COVID-19 pandemics can result in significant economic and social impacts that can take decades to reverse. The effects can manifest through many avenues, including job losses, commodity supply chain disruptions, significant drops in economic activity, poverty, and a rise in economic inequalities. On an individual level for households, the financial consequences may be seen through a loss of employment. Governments are very uncertain during these times as they are posed with the competing interests of allowing economic activities to continue as usual for the sake of the economy versus promoting and ensuring that its citizens have maximum protection against COVID-19.

The types of households can be divided into two broad categories, namely the poor and rich class. The poor are further classified into various categories, which determine their livelihoods and living standards. The households are thus classified as chronic poor, transient poor, vulnerable, middle class, and elite. The detailed discussions of the types of poverty fall outside the scope of this chapter, but it is sufficient to state that the sub-divisions simply help with the determination of propensity to either remain in or fall into poverty. Furthermore, categorization is vital as it aids in understanding the impact of a pandemic like COVID-19.

When one talks about poverty, reference is made to hunger and lack of shelter, illiteracy and not having access to school, being sick and unable to afford good medical care, fearing and being uncertain about the future. Examining this definition, poverty deals majorly with the standard of living of individuals and the ability to provide basic needs (Adefisoye & Adefisoye, 2020, pp. 15–31). Chen (2019) corroborated this and stated that poverty is a situation where people cannot afford the financial resources that can provide the resources to live above the minimum standard of living. Poverty affects every country in the world, but with different temerity and severances. Many people in Namibia still live in poverty and deplorable conditions. Some people do not have access to basic resources such as water and food, good sanitation, and accommodation.

Health Related Effects

The importance of health and medical care and medical knowledge cannot be overstated. According to estimates, life expectancy increased by several years before health and infectious disease mortality declined. Perhaps the greatest contribution that health and medical care can make is to raise the standard of living for those who are afflicted by disease (Rosen & Haglund, 2001, pp. 219–230). In Namibia, we have two primary health-care systems, namely private health care and the public known as the state health care system. The private health care system is believed to be better equipped with medical equipment and better services. Based on this assumption, private health care is more expensive and requires a patient to dig deeper into their pockets to enjoy services offered by such a system.

Conversely the state health care system is funded by the state and is therefore cheaper compared to the private health care system. Despite the belief that private health care system offers better services and medical treatment, Namibia has done well by ensuring that all its patients receive quality services at state hospitals. Ranging from primary health care to district hospitals, regional hospitals, intermediate hospitals, and the central hospital, the state offers medical care to all sorts of patients. Even though the state health care system provides good quality health care, poor persons and those from vulnerable groups do not have the choice to make use of private health care, which at times might provide better health care compared to its counterpart. Poor hygiene has adverse consequences on an individual and amplifies the transmission of pandemics such as COVID-19. Once a person who lives below the poverty line gets sick, he or she may not be able to afford proper healthcare. During this perilous time of COVID-19, many people lost their lives due to their inability to afford health care. Some Namibians live in rural areas far from towns where there are no proper hospitals, clinics, or healthcare institutions.

Employment Related Effects

The labor market of Namibia looks more vulnerable with unemployment increasing over the years, resulting in the rise of poverty and inequality. The number of people in employment declined over the past year, with the employment level now stands at 676,885 from 708,895 in 2014 (Financial Year 2020/2021 Budget Statement). One of the factors contributing to the rise in unemployment is the decrease in employment in the agricultural sector. Agricultural sector is one of the key sectors providing employment in Namibia, and any downscaling of employment in this sector will have severe consequences on the labor sector of Namibia (Financial Year 2020/2021 Budget Statement).

There are various factors that may be the cause of increasing unemployment, one of which is redundancy, which is the reduction of the workforce due to various structural and economic changes in an organization. Businesses made huge losses because of COVID-19. Although the pandemic affected all businesses across the board, the hospitality and the tourism industries have been affected the most. As a result of reduction in clientele and profit losses, most businesses have retrenched their employees. Seaflower Pelagic Processing company, Hilton Hotel, the Namibian Newspaper, Zelda Guest farm, Safari Hotel, and Canyon Hotel are some of the businesses that have retrenched workers in Namibia.

In terms of section 34 of the Labor Act, 11 of 2007, retrenchments may result from changes in the operational requirements or reduction of the workforce for economic or technical reasons. However, COVID-19-related retrenchments are mostly because of economic reasons. Businesses are losing huge amounts of money and are unable to maintain their wage bills, resultantly, retrenching some employees. Retrenched employees are heads of households and have dependents who are under their care both socially and financially. Thus, the increase in retrenchments country-wide results in a rise in unemployment and poverty.

Economic Related Effects

An Emergency Income Grant, providing a once-off payment of N$ 750 grant per person, was rolled out by costing the Government N$ 561.96 million

(Financial Year 2020/2021 Budget Statement). This Grant was meant to assist the low-income group, which was and continues to be very much affected by COVID-19. As much as this grant seemed to be a much-welcomed relief by those affected by the pandemic, it yielded very low results. It has fed the poor for a day, but it did not offer sustainable development to those affected. When an economy of a country falls, it is very difficult for such country to regain its economic freedom. A very clear example is our good neighbor Zimbabwe. During the rule of Robert Mugabe, Zimbabwe, which was once a rich country and an economic hub for Africa, now depends on foreign loans to make ends meet. The Zimbabwean currency has fallen, and the masses at the grassroot level are most affected by the status quo in Zimbabwe.

The Minister of Finance in his 2019/2020 budget speech revealed that a budget of N$ 727 million was frontloaded to the health sector. Mostly, such funds are required to procure medical equipment that can be used for the purposes of treating those affected by viruses. It is beyond debate that the lives of all Namibians are important and cannot be compared with money. However, do we need millions every time a pandemic hits to guarantee safety for Namibian citizens? Where have we lost principles of sustainable development? If all hospitals in Namibia, especially the state hospitals and facilities, were equipped with all medical equipment, even prior to the pandemic, would there be any need to pump large sums of money once off to treat patients affected by the virus? The Ministry of Health and Social Services has been receiving one of the biggest chunks of the national budget. Not discrediting the good done by the said Ministry over the years, the question remains: Has enough been done in our health sector, and is there still a need to pump millions or billions into the health sector?

National lockdowns and closure of borders to contain the virus have severe consequences on exports and imports. Trade between nations is one of the biggest contributors to the economic development of a country. The transfer of goods and services, including capital assets, between nations is referred to as international trade. Hence, to meet the requirements of people, businesses, and other businesses, international business consists of planned transactions that are carried out across national borders (Grozdanovskaa, Jankulovskib, & Bojkovska, 2017, pp. 105–114). When borders are closed to prevent any exit or entry into a country, exports and imports are controlled, which limits free trade. Although COVID-19 situation may require national lockdowns and closure of national borders, there is a need to perform a balancing act. The suggestion is not to compromise the health system. Rather, we need to balance how to protect the health of Namibians during the pandemic such as this whilst at the same time ensuring that economic activities continue. This is to avoid negatively affecting the livelihoods of the people, especially those in the informal sector.

Nationally, the lockdowns call for the closure of informal markets. Many unemployed Namibians put bread on the table with the income generated from such informal businesses. Once an informal business is closed as a result of state regulations, the vendors of informal businesses do not have any other source of income and may as a result not be in the position to take care of themselves. In Namibia, unemployment rate stood at 20.27 percent in 2019 and at 20.59 in 2020. Given the small population size, the numbers of the unemployed population rate is alarming.

POST-COVID-19 IMPLICATIONS

Namibia has been able to achieve upper-middle income status by reducing poverty and implementing strong economic policies since the attainment of independence in 1990. However, the COVID-19 pandemic only made socio-economic disparities worse, which are still a remnant of previous apartheid political systems. The generation of jobs has also been limited by structural growth restrictions. A relatively small segment of the population holds the economic advantage, and inequality continues. Large employees were laid off as companies struggled to maintain employment due to Namibia's weak economy, which was made worse by the COVID-19 pandemic. Most low-income employees, who are employed in manufacturing and construction businesses have been laid off and have no means of income as businesses in these industries continue to struggle to break even and guarantee good returns on their sales and provision of services. To push businesses into the "normal operational" mode, Namibian government has removed lockdowns and open up the business sector. It is believed that although this continues to assist with the recovery of the economic sector, it has also caused strain on the health sector as opening up of the economy contributed to the spread of COVID-19. During the outbreak of COVID-19, the government of Namibia was forced to implement measures to assist those struggling. One such measure was financial aid of 750 Namibian dollars given to each unemployed Namibian. In such instances, the government provided food parcels to the poor. All these measures caused a strain on the government as funds that could have been used for other developmental projects were injected into assisting the poor through quick help means. Since COVID-19, the government has lost out on millions as it helps to safeguard the economy of Namibia and provide means of survival to the poor. Namibia may have survived COVID-19, but the economic effects have continuously been experienced by the country. There is a need for a balanced approach of fighting COVID-19 on one hand and opening up the economy and promoting normal business activities on the other hand with the aim of turning the economy of the country..

CONCLUDING REMARKS

It is very clear that the actions of the apartheid government in Namibia have, to date, left Namibia with scars. Although Namibia has made efforts to deal with poverty, there is much that still needs to be done. The COVID-19 era in which we live has simply magnified the poverty and inequality in which many Namibians still find themselves. Persons in the informal sector and those in hospitality industries seem to be severely affected by the events of COVID-19. This is mainly because businesses in these sectors highly depend on physical contact with clients. Although the President has the power, in terms of his constitutional mandate under Article 26 of the Constitution, to declare a state of emergency and call for a national lockdown, it is very important that such be exercise taking into consideration its possible effects on the have-nots.

Corruption is one of the key enemies of our economy. Corruption causes the funds that could have been used for economic development programs to be diverted toward self-gain and self-gratification. Public funds should be used for purposes for which they have been allocated. Failing to do this will makc it impossiblc to promote the welfare of the people, as guaranteed in Article 95 of the Constitution. It is important for the Namibian government to put in place systems that will strongly monitor and combat corruption. A good corporate governance system becomes key in this instance. The government of Namibia should continuously partner with national and international organizations to invest more in the informal sector business. Without disputing the fact that some development has taken place in the information sector, the argument remains that not enough has been done and there is more to be done. If vendors in the informal sector become self-sufficient and are able to contribute meaningfully to the economy of the country, there will be no need for the government to pump huge amounts of money into this sector during difficult times such as COVID-19. Hence, time has come to think sustainable development.

REFERENCES

Adefisoye, Taiwo O., & Adefisoye, Ibironke D. COVID-19, Governments' Response and the Feminisation of Poverty: Ekiti State, Nigeria in Perspective. *Journal of Education Research and Rural Community Development*, 2, no. 1 (2020), 15–31.

Affirmative Action (Employment) Act, 1998 (Act 29 of 1998).

Compassion "Children and Poverty: What are the Main Causes of Poverty?" (2020). www.compassion.com/poverty/what-causes-poverty.htm, accessed 22 February 2022.

Constitution of Namibia.

Grozdanovskaa, V., Jankulovskib, N., & Bojkovska, K. International Business and Trade. *International Journal of Sciences: Basic and Applied Research*, 31, no. 3 (2017), 105–114.

Namibian Employers' Federation v President of the Republic of Namibia (HC-MD-CIV-MOT-GEN-2020/00136) [2020] NAHCMD 248 (23 June 2020).

Namibian Government: (Financial Year 2020/2021 Budget Statement).

New Economic Equitable Empowerment Framework (UN: Responsibility, Global and Solidarity-Responding to socio-economic impacts of COVID-19 March 2020).

Rosen, M., & Haglund, B. The Importance of Health and Medical Care for Public Health. *Scandinavian Journal of Public* Health, 29 (Suppl 58) (2001) 219–230.

The Namibian Newspaper http://www.namibian.com.na/6217119/archive-read/16-million-Namibians--living-in-poverty last, accessed 8 January 2023.

The World Bank in Namibia: https//www.worldbank.org/en/country/namibia/overview.

Chapter 9

The Impact of COVID-19 Pandemic on the Education System in Namibia

A Security Analysis

Monika Ndapandula Shifotoka and Abdallah Ally

INTRODUCTION

The World Health Organization (WHO) declared a global health concern on January 30, 2020, and on February 11, 2020, the coronavirus was assigned a scientific name COVID-19 (WHO, 2020). Public health information became significant to the public and a month later it was declared a world pandemic (Yue et al., 2020; Zu et al., 2020). Egypt was the first country in Africa that recorded its first case of the COVID-19 on February 14, 2020 (Gilbert et al., 2020; Anjorin, 2020).

Namibia recorded her first cases of infection on the March 14, 2020, and the Ministry of Education, Arts and Culture (MEAC) announced the closure of all public and private schools effectively on March 16, 2020 (UN Namibia, 2020), as a way of minimizing the spread of COVID-19. Other African countries did the same as the infection rates increased. Besides, some African countries faced challenges (Hopman, Allegranzi, & Mehtar, 2020). According to the United Nations Educational and Scientific Organization (UNESCO) 144 nations experienced country-wide closure of schools globally by the May 26, 2020. Countries such as China immediately put measures in place and kicked off online learning (Wang et al., 2020).

Not all nations had the necessary infrastructure and means of conducting online and distance learning. According to the International Telecommunications Union (ITU), though 89.4 percent of Africans have access to mobile-cellular network coverage, only 17.8 percent of households have internet access at home (ITU, 2020). Africa is one of the continents that has a low literacy rate, including disparities when it comes to access to internet and therefore a high in digital gap. There are several factors that should be considered when it comes to the impact that COVID-19 has on the education system. The challenges of online and distance learning that require technological infrastructure such as network coverage, access to computers and other gadgets, as well as the digital competencies and literacies. Other factors besides access are teachers' ability to adapt to delivering education remotely as it varies greatly considering the geographical location of a country. Not all teachers have the skills of planning lessons online due to long experience of teaching manually. Lastly, the increase in online activities without proper preparations means an increase in cyberattacks and online vulnerabilities. This section, therefore, aims to explore and identify potential effects of COVID-19 on education in Africa and proposes suggestions of how to mitigate the situation. Education is known to be the greatest equalizers in societies as it provides skills and competencies for the job market. It contributes to a knowledge-based economy and continuous learning. Education aid in conflict-affected countries is usually used to manage populations perceived as at risk. Education has the capacity to save and change lives. The prolonged closure of schools, therefore, has a risk of undermining aspirations and potential and sadly widening inequalities.

There have been several studies and literature on COVID-19 related to medical studies (Zu et al., 2020; Yue et al., 2020), but there is limited literature on COVID-19 and its hindrance to especially the education system in African context, a sector that is vital in every developing country. This section therefore contributes to literature through investigating the impact of COVID-19 on the education system, exploring strategies that were employed by schools in ensuring continuous delivery of quality education during this period, digital divide, and gap in learning. The chapter suggests strategies to be employed to mitigate the negative effects of COVID-19 to catch up adequately, especially for learners taking national examinations.

DIGITAL DIVIDE IN THE EDUCATION SYSTEM

There has been significant development and changes in the technological industry in the world, with countries such as Norway, Sweden, Netherlands, Denmark, the United States of America, and Singapore rising in terms of information, communication, technology, and innovation (Getzoff, 2020). These changes have ensured that the livelihoods of ordinary people are improved and services are brought closer to the people. The development of technology and digitization offers an environment where the public has access to free flow of information from large and diverse sources. Nevertheless, there has been a gap in terms of technological development, with some countries doing better than others. Statistics have indicated that Africa has a lot to do to catch up when it comes to digital divide that is seen through provincial and regional lens as well as gender gaps (Mutsvairo & Rognedda, 2019).

Gill and Karakülah (2018) argue that education, electricity, and taxes are Africa's three deadly deficits, with students in Sub-Saharan Africa having the lowest educational attainment. They further noted that lack of education is at the fundamental of most development problems. Lack of development in Africa and other developing countries has been a major challenge (Omotola, 2010). Nonetheless, countries have worked hard in ensuring that key aspects of society are put at the agenda of governments; furthermore, the adoption of the African Union Agenda for Development 2063 and the Sustainable Development Goals (SDGs) have striven to renew the drive for development in Africa.

The digital divide on the African continent usually resonances on gender, geographical location, race, and socioeconomic status (Mutsvairo & Rognedda, 2019). Therefore, several factors are considered when discussing the digital split. Digital divide is commonly defined, considering both access to and usage of information and communication technology (ICTs). Srinuan and Bohlin (2011) explain digital divide as the gap that separates those who have access to new types of ICTs from persons who do not have access and denote that digital divide can exist within a nation and between states. This gap is recognized as digital divide, which is amongst demographics and districts that have access to current information and communications technology and those that do not have restricted access (Sriruan & Bohlin, 2011). These technologies include gadgets, smartphones, computers, and the internet. Notwithstanding the progression made in technology, most learners in Africa are still not getting the benefits of these great technologies.

This is evident in many African countries, as indicated in a study by Sintema that revealed that due to limited technology resources, there are low levels of technology usage in secondary schools in Zambia (Sintema, 2020). Even though there has been significant improvement in internet connection, the African continent still records the lowest internet penetration rate of 39.3 percent (Internet World Statistics, 2020). The International Telecommunication Unit demonstrates a great broadband gap with few fixed broadband subscribers and mobile broadband subscriptions in Africa (Bagula, Zennaro, Nungu, & Nkoloma, 2011). This indicates the continuous rate of digital divide in Africa.

There are several causes of the digital divide, bearing in mind that the African continent is still developing and is underprivileged compared to most continents. Factors such as insufficient access to electricity and internet, affordability, lack of ICT infrastructure, limited access to internet, lack of technical support, mobile coverage, and technology at affordable costs. Additionally, most governments may not necessarily place ICT development at the core of the agenda, considering that there are other critical problems such as access to water, health care, housing, and other basic needs that may be priority than ICT development. Hagen (2007) argues that though it is vital to bridge digital divide on the continent, there are other challenges, such as political stability, that urgently need to be addressed.

Digital divide therefore became a hindrance during the times of COVID-19 as not all learners were able to access online learning. In most developing countries, telecommunications infrastructure may not be on the top of the agenda, and other development goals such as public health, shelter, access to water, and political stability have received higher priority, hence the increase in digital divide, which proved as a hindrance to the learning process during the COVID-19 pandemic as most of the learners were not able to learn online. Digital divide therefore became a hindrance during the times of COVID-19 as not all learners were able to access online learning.

ACCESS AND INFRASTRUCTURE

Governments, education departments, and schools attempted to conduct online learning for the learners; for example, the Namibian government through the MEAC, decided to implement online learning for public schools (Gervasius, 2020). The effort was to ensure that the learning process continued regardless of the pandemic. Hence, when it comes to online learning, one should consider access to the learning platforms. Certainly, it is agreeable that the internet plays a key role in facilitating good governance, improving education and health, transforming political processes, and strengthening participation in decision-making processes. It is important to build an inclusive society with free flow of information and strive to bridge the digital gap when it comes to internet and ICTs. The internet and new media technologies are helping to attain some of the essential goals of development. These goals include having an informed society, empowering communities, and democracy, in part through sharing information, participation in democratic discussions, online learning, e-commerce, and so forth.

Livingstone (2004) discusses that access to ICTs and media depends on dynamic and social process and is not a one-off piece of establishment. Once initial access is established, developing literacy leads users to alter significantly and continually the conditions of access, which include updating, upgrading, and extending hardware and software applications. Access means an opportunity to learn online and an opportunity for learners and students to practice what they have been taught, not only the theoretical part of ICTs. The poor and marginalized have always had historically poor access to communication tools and channels, and this is common in most developing countries (World Bank, UNESCO and UNICEF, 2021). Additionally, there is insufficient to technology, including connectivity to the internet, broadband, smart phones, gadgets, and unequal access to IT resources (Bomah, 2014). Those who are economically stable have the means to procure, get easy access to the newest technology, and acquire the best available learning aids. As a result, they excel in education, whereas those who do not have access to online learning will lag, increasing the disparity in learning. This additionally means that those who are disadvantaged will not be able to compete globally; therefore, lack of access due to COVID-19 reduces the chance of advancement in academic careers.

The implication is that there will be a socioeconomic development gap between individuals and societies prompted by the differences in the usage and development of ICTs (Bagula, Zennaro, Nungu, & Nkoloma, 2011). In other developing countries, such as China, close to one-half of the population has access to the internet and are active users (Qin, Stromberg, & Wu, 2017) due to technological development. Hence, Chinese universities responded quickly to COVID-19 challenges by means of utilizing innovative online education models (Wang, Cheng, Yue, & McAleer, 2020). This may not necessarily be the case in other parts of the world, including Africa. Electricity bills are typically high, and that poses a challenge for rural inhabitants. Moreover, electrical distributions of networks are poorly developed, which contributes to insufficient or lack of access as there are inadequate electrical power facilities to support ICT infrastructure in the rural areas. Developing countries have, in the last decade, been confronted with additional challenges of the emerging new information age. Even though there is a high penetration rate of mobile phones in developing countries, including Africa (Bagula, Zennaro, Nungu, & Nkoloma, 2011) not everyone will necessarily have a smart phone. Just as every innovation brings both opportunities and challenges, the technology in the education industry has its own challenges.

There are inequalities in terms of access to technology and resource distribution and skills required for individuals to efficiently participate in the digital environment. Furthermore, one should comprehend the impact of technology on education during the time of COVID-19 as a result affecting the way education is delivered. Nonetheless, there is a gap in access to the internet between rich and poor, especially those from disadvantage backgrounds leading to high inequalities in educational success in developing countries. Consequently, it is vital that educators be aware of the potential barriers to technology and internet access that learners may face. Digital divide remains in societies and limits the participation of people in the digital era in a variety of ways, such as the affordability of users, willingness to participate, digital and English literacies. Many internet users lack English language and prerequisites to use the internet (Srinuan & Bohlin, 2011). Even though online content is available in other languages as well, most of the texts are mostly in English, which may not be understood by everyone, especially by parents and guardians who are supposed to guide, supervise, and check for their children's progress during this period.

The internet environment has advanced with social media becoming popular globally, and because of its prospective enormous role it became immensely popular. Individuals in different countries utilize some of these platforms, such as WhatsApp and WeChat, to share learning materials; however, not everyone, especially pupils, may have access to a smartphone, and internet connection access can also be a hindrance. COVID-19 has greatly affected the learning process as there has been a loss of contact hours for learners and students and lack of e-learning facilities that might be used for teaching purposes (Sintema, 2020). While some may consider postponement of the school calendar, chances are that education ministries, departments, and councils may not necessarily postpone the writing of national examinations, meaning there is a possibility that learners might not be well equipped and ready for these exams. Learners and students in remote areas without access to proper network coverage will also miss out on the opportunity of learning. The gap between rich and poor plays a role, as those from poor backgrounds may not necessarily be able to afford smartphones and gadgets.

Education is a basic human right in countries such as Namibia, where it is enshrined in chapter 3, article 20 in the Namibian Constitution (Namibian constitution, 2019). It enables people to get knowledge and acquire skills, which in turn empowers people; therefore, it will be unfair that some pupils are not able to continue learning to hindrance of access and infrastructure when it comes to ICTs. It is important to point out the different classes in society; therefore, not all learners and students have access to technology or a suitable learning environment at home, as they had to go back home to villages and rural areas. The digital divide illustrates that access to internet and mobile network differs significantly in low-income countries; therefore, online learning will be easier for individuals with access and will exclude a sizeable number of disadvantaged learners. These learners may not have electricity, internet, and Wi-Fi connections; some do not have computers and televisions at home; others will have basic-feature mobile phones but not necessarily smartphones; and others will have only little bandwidth and internet connection. Other challenges include broadband internet availability and limited access to free community internet in public buildings (Ramset & Adams, 2020). Changes in technology such as the tools and platforms that are being used can also play a role. Affordability of devices such as laptops, tablets, and smartphones, inability to operate and work with proposed learning programs.

Therefore, lack of access and infrastructure played a big role and are a hindrance to the continuous learning environment because of COVID-19, hence disturbing the learning process as online and e-learning were not successfully implemented. COVID-19 has made noticeable the inequalities that already exist in our societies. These concerns threaten to leave a fragment of learners and students even further behind their peers in education achievement.

DIGITAL LITERACY IN EDUCATION

Defeating digital divide and having access to ICTs does not necessarily mean that people are able to use them effectively; in fact, one may have access to all these technologies, but they do not necessarily have the competencies and know-how of operating the platforms and gadgets. This is another hindrance to the learning process during the pandemic. Hutchinson (2016) noted that it is challenging to establish systems, digital tools, and methodologies at the same rate with connected devices and connect emerging research practices with a media and communication perspective (Hutchinson, 2016). Even those who may have access to the internet and ICTs the question is: are they able to utilize these tools effectively? It is, therefore, significant that the promotion of digital and media literacy is advanced. Digital literacy has been defined as "the ability to understand and use information in multiple formats from a wide variety of sources when it is presented via computers and particularly through the medium of the internet" (Gilster, in Pool, 1997, 6). One should acquire the competencies and skills to utilize platforms and comprehend data that is available online. Gilster classified knowledge assembly, evaluating information content, searching the internet, and navigating hypertext as some of the major digital literacy competencies (Gilster, 1997).

It is vital that online users are able to not only access technology and new media but also evaluate, understand, and utilize these online tools. A study conducted in schools in Cape Town, South Africa, discovered that digital equity has not been reached when learners ICT competence is compared even though all schools employ ICT in their curriculum (Gudmundsdottir, 2010). It should be clear that being digitally literate can empower citizens to be able to create their own content and participate in online discussions. This is a demonstration of the challenges that the education system is facing when it comes to especially digital divide. Digital literacy is directly affected by restricted resources and budgets, as well as the unqualified teachers in this field, training for the trainers and the incorporation and implementation of media and information literacy into the education curricula, which is an important element for any social development. This is revealing that when it comes to online learning, there are many factors to consider and lack of understanding of digital media and information literacy from both teachers and learners may all hinder effective learning process. The challenge with digital gap is that it is not just about giving someone a smartphone or gadget but having the competencies of utilizing it; therefore, the aspects connectivity and functionality of the devices are also important.

EDUCATION AND SECURITY

Security is vital and should be considered when it comes to the impact of COVID-19 on education. Due to the unexpected closure of school's facilities, management did not plan on how they would handle risks that can be brought about by online learning, such as cyberattacks; hence, without any warning for institutions to prepare, COVID-19 has made cyber security more complicated. Just like governments and health professionals need to be able to monitor disease hot spots and high-risk areas, IT technicians and cyber security managers are also supposed to monitor and ensure that they can understand where to focus their resources, enforce policies, and mitigate online risks and vulnerabilities.

Threat actors such as hackers have many opportunities to gain a grip, more so now as there has been a huge flow in the remote workforce. Since teachers and other educational administrators worked remotely, their digital attack surface vastly expanded their networks and became vulnerable online users, as using school devices and digital tools will increase visibility online. Those who accessed systems outside the school premises may invite hackers, as there is no proper protection against viruses and online vulnerabilities. These networks present unique potential exposures and vulnerabilities, and hackers will continue to look for new ways to exploit fear and vulnerabilities. One of the biggest challenges is getting fact time with a school's IT department, who are instrumental in the deployment of any new IP-based security solution in an educational setting since COVID-19 has caused widespread closures of classrooms and other school buildings. Due to the closure of schools, children are expected to use laptops, mobile phones, and other gadgets to access e-learning and complete tasks.

This has increased the amount of time that they spend online and unsupervised content, which can be disadvantage as it will increase online bullying, expose users to child pornography, and other online vulnerabilities. Additionally, most home networks do not have internet security such as firewalls, which increases cyberattacks. Hackers take advantage of the fact that children do not always know about digital security, and if parents are overwhelmed and distracted, they may not be able to monitor their children's online activities. Information security is crucial, and it is important that there is safe flow of personal data and the protection of children online and their digital rights, as more children are online than ever. The pandemic may therefore have amplified children's vulnerability online.

The education and promotion of usage of ICTs and digital literacy competencies will make learners especially aware of online risks such as data protection and child pornography and how they can be vigilant while using the internet. Additionally, cyber security leaders, information technology technicians, and school management should prepare for how to educate children and teachers about safety in an online space. Once there is a threat to the education of a nation than the economy and other sectors of the country is affected; therefore, education is key to national security. Learners that were enrolled in science and information technology will be the cybersecurity experts tomorrow and will protect the nation from cyberattacks. Those enrolled in biology and research could develop medical cures tomorrow; therefore, any negative disruption to education is a threat to the security of any nation.

REPERCUSSIONS OF COVID-19 ON THE EDUCATION SYSTEM

Accessibility and Connectivity

While in some societies learners rely on e-learning, unfortunately, in most African countries, learners do not attend classes due to challenges in terms of accessibility and connectivity. Unlike other parts of world where colleges and universities have executed online learning platforms to assist teachers with conducting online lectures through systematic training and technical support (Wang, Cheng, Yue, & McAleer, 2020). Teachings were delivered through Tencent meetings and Zoom applications to ensure that those in different parts of the country and world have access to learning materials. This is, however, different in African countries where there are challenges of access, infrastructure, and other factors when it comes to online learning. This increases inequality in the learning process and threatens prospects and opportunities for these learners.

Digital Literacy and ICT Skills

A study by Sintema (2020) with secondary school teachers revealed that there is a possibility of the pass rate dropping during the national examination because of COVID-19 pandemic. This is due to the disruption of learning since the untimely closure of schools nationally. Teachers may not necessarily have the required competencies to prepare teaching materials and conduct online learning. Many countries have resulted to distance learning. However, these are means that may not be practical considering that not all learners may have access to internet or gadgets such as smartphones and computers. Unfortunately, pupils, especially in rural areas, live distances apart from schools; therefore, it may not also be practical to physically distribute educational materials to all pupils and students. Hence, the learners and parents are not able to collect reading materials during the time of lockdown and do not have access to smartphones so that they receive the reading materials online, further making it difficult for continuous learning during the period of lockdown due to the pandemic. Even though learning resources may be available, it might be challenging ensuring that all pupils have access to them. This may widen equity gaps as some pupils will be left out. Access to electricity is the biggest challenge in Africa. Even though renewable energies like solar energy are promising solutions to meet the need for electricity, especially in rural households and community centers in remote locations (Bagula, Zennaro, Nungu, & Nkoloma, 2011), it is still a challenging factor as the general population does not have access to electricity, meaning that it is challenging for people to charge their phones and access other services that require electricity and power.

Delivering Quality Education

Teachers had to be creative and come up with strategies that could strengthen and enhance quality teaching. This can be overwhelming, especially if there is no proper support from either school management or government. Additionally, not all teachers may have the capacity and skills to use online teaching resources and tools such as Google Classroom, Skype, and Zoom meetings. The massive digital divide in the education system means it is a hindrance to the development of especially underdeveloped areas. Pupils and students are even more disadvantaged when it comes to subjects that require practicals and laboratories, as there is no means of actually getting in the premises. Online exams are also limited in terms of hours that are allocated, as perhaps the institutions fears that students will copy. At the end of the day, during tests and examinations, time is too limited, making it challenging for students to finish writing on time. Considerations from schools and institution of high learning on refunds as pupils and students were away basically paying for some of the services that were not provided. Most students and pupils live in the villages and farms where there is no access to internet.

Educational Services

In addition, school is not only a place for learning and studying; however, that is where most of the children get a warm meal, which was also encouraging the children to come to school. Additionally, learners from disadvantageous backgrounds and communities, refugees, and children with disabilities may also be greatly affected, as they might not be included in planning and sometimes have lower educational outcomes than their peers. Similarly, we foresee a higher rate of learners drop out from schools as a result of this enormous disruption to access to education.

IMPACT OF COVID-19 ON THE EDUCATION SYSTEM IN NAMIBIA

Government Response to COVID-19

Article 20 of the Namibian constitution states that all persons shall have the right to education. This means that governments are supposed to provide facilities to ensure access to learning, as lack of access to online learning can impact on the right to education. In response to reduce the spread of the virus, the President of the Republic of Namibia declared a state of emergency as stipulated in article 26 (1) of the Namibian Constitution. The MEAC announced the closure of all public and private schools in the country with immediate effect from March 16, 2020, which was for both learners and teachers. This also included the College of the Arts, libraries, Resource Centers, Museums etc. Schools with hostels countrywide embarked on deciding for learners to leave schools without further infections. The school calendar was amended; therefore, learners did not receive their first-term progress report, and evaluation was set to be done in the second term to cover the curriculum for both first and second terms. The re-opening of the schools was slated for the April 14, 2020, and the school managements were cautioned to ensure that the schools were clean and safe for the return of learners. Due to COVID-19, the education sector has been pushed to change. The country has witnessed unexpected breakthroughs, with some schools quickly embracing platforms like WhatsApp, including other modes like Google Classroom and Zoom (Siririka, 2020).

Parents and guardians were tasked to oversee and supervise learners at home with regards to ensuring that their schoolwork is completed in the required time. Additionally, they were requested to ensure that appropriate precautionary measures are taken at home to ensure that their children are practicing hygiene through washing hands and other means in order to minimize the spread of the virus. Due to the increase in cases and considering the safety of learners and teachers, the re-opening of schools was postponed to June 3, 2020, when Namibia resumed face-to-face classes for senior secondary grades 11 and 12 after the lockdown. The schools were advised to adhere to practicing social distancing and safety hygiene measures to curb the spread of the virus.

School Closures Consequences

COVID-19 affected education through temporary closures and disruptions in learning in an attempt to slow the spread of the virus. This, however, disadvantaged learners and students as there was a lack of student-teacher interaction that can lead to students and learners feeling demotivated, uninspired, and less passionate about their schoolwork. Hence, some learners and students may not put in much effort in school. School closures also meant that learners no longer had access to school feeding programs, which motivated some learners to attend school. Those from disadvantaged backgrounds may not have the parental support needed to learn on their own. Opportunities for development were also minimized as learners could not take part in essay competitions and other initiatives that are available at schools.

Access to Information and Communication Technologies (ICTs)

In seeking to minimize the potential transmission, MEAC called for the implementation of virtual learning. Nonetheless, lack of access to ICTs and fast and reliable internet connections can be a hindrance and prevent learners and students especially, those from villages and areas without proper internet connect to access education during this period. Learners and students may not complete tasks on time as they do not have access to internet at home. The closures of school libraries increased the difficulty of keeping up with online learning, as those dependent on the library for internet access could not do that. Technology can enable teachers, learners, students, and parents to access materials and continue learning. However, access, digital and media literacy skills, online supervisor, teacher-learner participation hinder online learning. UNESCO (2020) recommended the use of distance learning programs and platforms that can be utilized to reach learners and students remotely while minimizing the disruption of education; however, the ultimate closure of schools did not give educators and planners enough time to strategize on best practices, especially in the early stages of the pandemic.

ACCESS TO EDUCATIONAL RESOURCES

Closure of schools and disruption in learning meant that not much access was provided to textbooks and materials provided by teachers and librarians. Even though learners could not access books and materials via the library, teachers were also challenged to access resources for online teaching and to share them with their learners. Since there was no proper planning with regard to online and distance learning, some teachers may not have the necessary skills to access information from open educational resources and needed training on online teaching, copyright issues with regard to the online resources, and how to navigate the e-learning systems.

Effective Teaching and Quality Education

The closure of schools also affected students' and learners' learning outcomes. Teachers were challenged to deliver quality education and pressed to finish the syllabus and curriculum without properly planning on best practices and considering challenges faced by learners. Parents and guardians were tasked to facilitate and supervise online and distance learning of children at home. They may be challenged, overwhelmed, and struggle to take up this task considering that some parents have limited educational backgrounds and not all are equipped for homeschooling.

SURVEY ON THE IMPACT OF COVID-19 ON THE EDUCATION SYSTEM IN NAMIBIA

As part of getting information about the reality on the ground, an online survey was administered to teachers that work for the MEAC. Data was collected from 12 teachers at Windhoek High School, Khomas Region, and 14 teachers Kuisebmund Secondary School, Erongo Region, for a total of 25 teachers completing the online survey. Microsoft Forms were used to design the questionnaire, and a link was distributed to teachers via WhatsApp. The two schools were selected as the ones that the researcher had access to. The following are the questions and summary of the answers from the respondents.

Strategies that Teachers and Schools Utilized

The respondents indicated several strategies that they utilized to ensure continuous learning for students, regardless of the pandemic. They had to reduce the number of students in their classes as a way of practicing social distancing for key grades such as grade 11 and grade 12 as they had to continue with physical classes. Teachers indicated that they compiled materials and sent to parents and learners via social media platforms such as WhatsApp for those who had access to computers, mobile phones, internet, and other ICT gadgets; therefore, activity handouts were given to learners to work on during lockdown. Additionally, some teachers attempted to phone the parents and encouraged them to visit the schools and collect the materials, especially those who did not have access to the internet. Applications such as WhatsApp, Google Classroom and Zoom were used for students who had access to the internet. Unfortunately, some teachers indicated that they did not conduct any classes during this time and did not make any special arrangements for the learners.

Effect of COVID-19 Learners' Performance in the National Examination

There is a consensus among the teachers on the negative effect of the pandemic and closure of schools on the quality of education. According to the respondents, they will have to cover a lot of information from the syllabus in a short period of time, which may be overwhelming, especially to learners; hence, some teachers indicated that they are not confident that they will be able to cover all the content in the syllabus. Additionally, learners will not be taught effectively considering the time that has been lost due to the closure of schools and that they foresee poor performance, especially those who will write the national examination. Some indicated that learners have switched off emotionally from school and it will be difficult for them to catch up with limited time left. Also, there is no proper supervision from teachers to ensure students are doing their schoolwork, and there are some parents who are not able to be involved in the education of their children, either that they are illiterate or do not have the skills or time.

Slow learners will be affected the most, said one of the respondents that it will be difficult for those academically challenged to be on pair with others. One respondent suggested that the school calendar be postponed to 2021 as it might be difficult to successfully complete this year's school activities and syllabus. However, some teachers are optimistic that if learners, teachers, and schools work together and through team effort, they can still be able to revise and dedicate time to assisting learners when schools resume. They are dedicated to ensuring that learners catch up with what they have missed.

Teachers' Challenges During the COVID-19 Period

Generally, lack of access to the internet came out as the biggest challenge faced by teachers; they also indicated that they received complaints from parents that they do not have access. Additionally, the lack of physical interaction with learners was detrimental to the learning process, since learning occurred on digital platforms and only few learners could afford to access these digital platforms..

Practices for Online Teaching

The respondents suggested that the usage of Google Classroom, WhatsApp, and Zoom platforms would be ideal if most learners had access to them. They indicated that they are supposed to create a supportive learning environment for learners by engaging with them online and urged the government to invest in infrastructure development to ensure that all people have access to the internet. Since it will take a while for the implementation of online learning, it is suggested that teachers and subject coordinators work together to come up with alternative learning besides online, as currently it is not a viable solution. One of the respondents suggested that the government provide a tablet for each learner so that they can implement online and digital learning. Another suggested schools should create websites that have learning materials and educate parents and learners on how to utilize it effectively. They are also advocating for all schools to have access to the internet and teachers should have access to parents' mobile numbers to communicate and look at how best they can send materials for the learners. A recommendation was made for the Ministry of Education to design a central system for dissemination of same information for each grade countrywide. Radio and television were indicated as the best means of communication, as most learners and parents have access to them. Teachers training on how to use e-learning and online applications. E-learning was identified as the most challenging to implement in public schools.

Strategies to Mitigate Negative Effects of COVID-19

The respondents indicated that they will be giving extra classes, ensuring that learners have access to past examination papers, revision before examinations, study sessions for hostel learners, and extra classes will be given during weekends and holidays. They will pay special attention to grade 11 and 12 learners and will encourage parents to monitor and motivate their children to study hard. Moreover, they will create notes that are learner and parents friendly that can be printed for the learners, especially those who do not have access to the internet, revising with learners that have access to the internet. One respondent called for the suspension or postponement of the 2020 academic and school years.

Digital Divide and Effect on Education

Learners in rural areas and those who do not have access to internet are completely left out and are not able to learn during this period; hence, digital gap illustrated how the MEAC is not prepared for online learning, and it is especially unfair for the students from disadvantaged backgrounds. Additionally, some students may have access to the internet but do not possess ICT tools. The respondents indicated that it would take a while for the country to move from the traditional way of learning to digital learning. The consensus is that learners from disadvantaged backgrounds were severely affected by the closure of schools as they were not able to access learning materials.

POST-COVID-19 IMPLICATIONS

Schools were reopened after months of lockdown, but the process was not easy. Some parents were hesitant to send their kids back to school because they were concerned that if there were no safeguards in place to stop the spread of COVID-19, their kids might get sick. The education system has been forced to discover alternative methods of teaching and learning by utilizing latest online teaching approaches because of the COVID-19 pandemic.

As a result of COVID-19, Namibia's media mix for learning now includes radio, television, print media, SMS, and social media, as well as both third-party and government-created learning platforms. The Namibia Reads app, which is accessible on Android and iOS devices, has also received promotion from the MEAC. Reading and learning are made simple for parents and kids with the help of this educational software for kids, which features an exclusive library of Real Along instructional books for kids ages 2 to 11. It benefits parents by helping their kids prepare ready for preschool and kindergarten, as well as advance in elementary school. This is one of the innovations that came from the pandemic and will continue to assist both learners and parents even after the pandemic. To deliver remote education at scale, Rodriguez et al. (2020) emphasized arranging education systems for learning recovery and putting innovative coping practices into practice. He argued that educational systems must create strategies for enhancing and quickening the learning process.

As a result of the closure of schools and the postponement and cancellation of exams, Namibia and other regions of the African continent saw a disruption in the progress made in attaining access to education. Most teachers and students in the nation are still learning about e-learning and online education in general, and many lack the tools and infrastructure needed to teach and study online (Bruno et al., 2020). An ethnographic narrative of the learning design experiences of six Namibian teachers during school closures brought on by the COVID-19 pandemic was presented in a study by (Boer & Asino, 2022).

The findings showed that teacher ICT competence and confidence, as well as a lack of infrastructure, access, and connectivity, had an impact on decisions concerning learning design. The teachers also emphasized that a stronger understanding of how to produce learning materials generally should be a focus for professional development in addition to ICT skills and creating learning materials for an online platform (Boer & Asino, 2022). The future of Namibia's educational system depends on the swift adoption of ICT, and COVID-19 is the catalyst for this adoption. Education must heavily rely on technology in the post-COVID era for both delivery and learning. To prepare students for employment in fields where technology is widely used, updated educational curricula should include teaching digital and social/emotional skills to students. Though the pandemic disrupted the learning situation in the country, one can argue that COVID-19 served as an enabler for the improvement of online learning and teaching in the Namibian education system.

RECOMMENDATIONS

Due to the rapid closures of schools, little or not much was done in planning for distance and online learning on the potential threats that it will bring to both the pupils and teachers. Authorities should consult teachers so that they discuss how they could provide materials and education to their pupils; they should be encouraged to share ideas and solutions that work best for them and require low-tech solutions such as communication via SMS, as the shutting down of schools and universities caused by the pandemic is making it more difficult for vulnerable students to receive quality education.

Governments and schools should adopt school policies that deal with crisis situations that could be implemented in future in similar cases. These policies should address the issue of ICTs and digital divide and design practical strategies for ensuring the continuity of learning and access to quality education regardless of circumstances. The challenge was attempting to virtually educate students for months on end when a significant portion of them don't have the internet access and computers they need to effectively do their work. Therefore, the school systems should be prepared to come up with structures that will assist with dealing with these situations in future.

Instead of focusing on individual access to the internet, African countries could instead explore a possibility of looking at how it can provide internet access to communities through centers like multi-purpose community centers and public libraries. Access to the internet needs to be equalized and appropriate tools and applications need to be established so all members of all societies can benefit from the digital revolution.

Teachers and school management should receive more support to ensure that they continue educating the African child, no matter the circumstances. There are some pupils who are already struggling to have enough schoolbooks, and the gap increases as they are expected to have internet access to take part in the online learning. Hence, it is vital that those at the forefront of planning in the MEAC in Namibia strategize to ensure that there are alternatives to deliverance of quality education. In Namibia, for example, some schools have utilized communication with parents through WhatsApp or SMS on a weekly basis by giving instructions on what the pupil should learn. However, this method is challenging as not all parents and guardians may have smartphones or do not have sufficient time to ensure that their children's activities are completed. Consequently, it means that homeschooling may not necessarily be ideal considering that most of the population does not have access to a laptop or home-based internet as per the International Telecommunication Union (ITU, 2020). UNESCO (2020) recommended the usage of low-technology platforms and applications as well as the usage of distance learning programs that reach learners remotely while still minimizing the disruption of education.

Radio is still Africa's most important source of information, with countries such as Namibia, Mali, and South Africa still relying on radio despite more digital offerings. What is challenging is how people listen to radio, as they can do that through mobile phones and internet (Wilhelm & Lorgerie, 2020). Most households in Sub-Saharan Africa have radio programs remains to make more than half of broadcasters output as it is produced cheaply, is affordable to consumers and reaches the disadvantage people faster (Wilhelm & Lorgerie, 2020). Ministries and departments of education, in collaboration with teachers, can create educational content that could be delivered through radio and television, as they are still important tools of communication on the continent and are easily accessible to most of the population. Learners and teachers should educate on the basic issues of online protection, risks and cybersecurity principles, such as using firewall for their internet connection, downloading and installing software updates as they become available, installing and regularly updating antivirus software's for computers and laptops, regular change of passwords, securing Wi-Fi networks, and so on. The aim is for users to know about the opportunities and as well as the risks of using ICT tools and platforms so that they are empowered to protect their data. Additionally, ministries of education should strive to incorporate, implement, and promote teaching of digital literacy through the formal curriculum to provide skills and competencies that will empower learners and teachers to be vigilant online.

CONCLUSION

COVID-19 has negatively impacted different sectors and changed the way in which teachers conduct teaching. Learners and teachers had to start utilizing online tools due to social distancing and closure of schools, resulting in a disparity in the provision of education. Lack of infrastructure, access, digital divide, and cyberattacks are some of the key challenges that the education system faced during the closure of schools. Those from disadvantaged and poor backgrounds were not able to learn during this period, so they will be lagging when the classes resume.

Clearly COVID-19 global pandemic has negatively impacted the education system, and the closure and disruption in learning will not only be felt in the national examination results; however, it will have long-term implications for the education system in Namibia, Africa, and globally. The impact might continue as there is no clear indication of how long the virus will be around, which means further disruption in the learning process. In countries such as Kenya, the government has indefinitely postponed the opening of the schools to the next academic year, which is 2021, and encouraged homeschooling. However, it should be noted that not many parents can afford and have expertise to homeschool their children, hence questioning the implications it will have for quality education.

Due to difficulties such as limited or lacking skills, resources, connectivity, and infrastructure; technology resistance and apathy by students, teachers, and parents; public schools not equipped for online learning, increasing the risk of learners falling behind; and not having enough time to implement and measure the impact of initiatives, teachers' forced migration to digital learning and teaching was very difficult.

The Namibian government and other developing countries need to explore new ways of expanding information infrastructure and increasing access to ICTs by reducing the cost of service, especially when it comes to access to computers and internet. Hence, it is vital that governments and the IT industry provide cost-effective and affordable services for people. Promoting digital literacy is very vital through campaigns or incentives and forming partnerships with successful entities. Investing in internet access means that the continent can build on the digitization transformation that is mostly needed and adjust with the changes that have been brought by the pandemic to ensure for continuous learning of students. Lastly, education departments should ensure they have plans that will deal with disruptions in the normal provision of education and look at implementing practical learning that will not further create disparities and inequalities in learning. Schools should invest in the promotion of digital literacy to create awareness about violations of privacy and risks associated with online learning and security. Learners have the prospects of becoming doctors, engineers, entrepreneurs, researchers, and scientists. Ensuring access to education during times of national disruption is vital, as education is key to national security.

Countries should develop frameworks and policies to be implemented to help countries mitigate and manage similar situations that will ensure continuity in education. A review revealed that most of the metrics used to understand well-being were imported from western contexts; their application did not fit rural Africa (Amina & Keevy, 2022). It is crucial that governments and schools create and implement culturally relevant initiatives that fit the context of certain regions. Though COVID-19 disrupted the education system, it has also opened opportunities to accelerate ICT integration into the education systems in Namibia and Africa as a whole.

REFERENCES

Amina, O., & Keevy, J. (2022). The Impact of COVID 19 on Education Systems in the Commonwealth. Commonwealth Secretariat. https://doi.org/10.14217/ComSec.950.

Anjorin, A. A. (2020). "The Coronavirus Disease 2019 (COVID 19) Pandemic: A Review and an Update on Cases in Africa". *Asian Pacific Journal of Tropical Medicine*, 13(5), 199–203. https://doi.org/10.4103/1995-7645.281612.

Bagula, A., Zennaro, M., Nungu, A., & Nkoloma, M. (2011, October). "Bridging the Digital Divide in Africa: A Technology Perspective". *Wireless Communication and Information (WCI 2011) on Digital Divide and Mobile Applications*. Retrieved from https://www.researchgate.net/publication/233817849.

Barron-Rodriguez, M., Cobo, C., Munoz-Najar, A., & Sanchez-Ciarrusta, I. (2021). Remote Learning during the Global Lockdown: Multi-Country Lessons (English). Washington, D.C., World Bank Group. https://doi.org/10.1596/36141

Boer, P. J., & Asino, T. I. (2022). "Learning Design Experiences of the Namibian Teachers during the COVID 19 Pandemic: An Ethnographic Perspective". *TechTrends*, 66, 29–38. https://doi.org/10.1007/s11528-021-00684-8.

Bomah, K. B. (2014, December). "Digital Divide: Effects on Education Development in Africa". YIT Dept. of Computing: Technical Writing Presentation, Ireland. Retrieved from https://www.researchgate.net/publication/275350414.

Chalita, S., & Erik, Bohlin. (2011, September 18). "Understanding the Digital Divide: A Literature Survey and Ways Forward". 22nd European Regional Conference of the International Telecommunications Societys, Budapest. Retrieved from http://hdl.handle.net/10419/52191.

Ester Mbathera. (2022, January 27). Covid 19 Continues to Shake Up Education Sector. Spotlight on Education. *The Namibian Newspaper* (p4). https://www.namibian.com.na/public/uploads/documents/61f38fe742abe/spotlight-on-education.pdf.

Gervasius, N. (2020). "Compulsory E-learning in Namibia's Public Schools: A Commendable Idea Marred by Digital Divide?". African Declaration on Internet Rights and Freedoms. Retrieved from https://africaninternetrights.org/en/updates/compulsory-e-learning-namibia's-public-schools-commendable-idea-marred-digital-divide.

Getzoff, M. (2020, January 17). Most Technologically Advanced Countries in the World 2020. Global Finance. Retrieved from https://www.gfmag.com/global-data/non-economic-data/best-tech-countries.

Ghebreyesus, D. T. A. (2020). Statement on the Second Meeting of the International Health Regulations (2005) Emergency Committee Regarding the Outbreak of Novel Coronavirus (2019-nCoV). Retrieved from https://www.who.int/emergencies/diseases/novel-coronavirus-2019/media-resources/press-briefings.

Gilbert, M., Pullano, G., Pinotti, F., Valdano, E., Poletto, C., Boëlle, P.-Y., D'Ortenzio, E., Yazdanpanah, Y., Eholie, S. P., Altmann, M., Gutierrez, B., Kraemer, M., & Colizza, V. (2020). "Preparedness and Vulnerability of African Countries against Importations of COVID 19: A Modelling Study". *The Lancent*, 395(10227), 871–877. http://doi.org/10.1016/S0140-6736(20)30411-6.

Gilster, P. (1997). *Digital Literacy*. New York: Wiley Computer Publications.

Global Monitoring of School Closures Caused by Covid 19. (2020, May 25). Retrieved from https://en.unesco.org/covid19/educationresponse.

Gudmundsdottir, G. (2010). "From Digital Divide to Digital Equity: Learners' ICT Competence in Four Primary Schools in Cape Town, South Africa". *International Journal of Education and Development Using Information and Communication Technology*, 6(2), 84–105. https://doi.org/10.1080/02681102.2010.498409.

Hagen, E. (2007). *The Digital Divide in Africa*. VDM Verlag Dr. Mueller e.K.

Hopman, J., Allegranzi, B., & Mehtar, S. (2020). "Managing COVID 19 in Low- and Middle-Income Countries". *JAMA*. https://doi.org/10.1001/jama.2020.4169.

Hutchinson, J. (2016). "An Introduction to Digital Media Research Methods: How to Research and the Implications of New Media Data". *Communication, Research and Practice*, 2(1), 1–6.

International Telecommunication Union. (2020). "Measuring Digital Development: Facts and Figures" (2020). Retrieved December 10, 2020 from https://www.itu.int/en/ITU-D/Statistics/Pages/facts/default.aspx on 5 December 2020.

International Telecommunication Union (ITU). (2020). Measuring Digital Development: Facts and Figures 2020. Retrieved from https://www.itu.int/en/ITU-D/Statistics/Pages/facts/default.aspx on 5 December 2020.

Kellner, D., & Share, J. (2007). "Critical Media Literacy is not an Option". *Learning Inquiry*, 1, 59–69. https://doi.org/10.1007/s11519-007-0004-2.

Lauren Mueenuddin. (2021, January). RTA of UNICEF's Ongoing Response to COVID 19: Nambia. Oxford Policy Management. https://www.unicef.org/esa/media/8566/file/RTA-Phase1-Nambia.pdf.

Livingstone, S. (2004). "Media Literacy and the Challenge of New Information and Communication Technologies". *The Communication Review*, 7, 3–14. https://doi.org/10.1080/10714420490280152.

Mare, A. (2018). "New Media Technologies and Internal Newsroom Creativity in Mozambique". *Digital Journalism*, 2(1), 12–28. https://doi.org/10.1080/21670811.2013.850196.

Mutsvairo, B., & Ragnedda, M. (2019). *Mapping the Digital Divide in Africa.* Amsterdam University Press.

Nampresidency. (2020). Statement by H.E. President Hage G. Geingob following Confirmation of Two Cases of COVID 19 on Namibian Soil 14 March 2020. Retrieved from https://op.gov.na/statements on 10 December 2020.

Omotola, Jeremiah Shola. (2010). "The Challenges of Development in Africa: Globalisation and New Regionalism". *World Affairs: The Journal of International Issues*, 14(2), 22–46. https://www.jstor.org/stable/48505058.

Pool, C. R. (2007). "A New Digital Literacy: A Conversation with Paul Gilster". *Educational Leadership*, 55(3), 6–11.

Qin, B., Strömberg, D., & Wu, Y. (2017). "Why Does China Allow Freer Social Media? Protests versus Surveillance and Propaganda". *Journal of Economic Perspectives*, 31(1), 117–140. https://doi.org/10.1257/jep.31.1.117.

Ramsetty, A., & Adams, C. (2020). "Impact of the Digital Divide in the Age of COVID 19". *Journal of the American Medical Informatics Association.* https://doi.org/10.1093/jamia/ocaa078.

Shelleygan Petersen. (2022, January 27). Virtual Learning: The New Normal for Schools?. The *Namibian Newspaper* (P3). https://www.namibian.com.na/public/uploads/documents/61f38fe742abe/spotlight-on-education.pdf.

Shikololo, A. (2020, 15 April). The Ministry of Education Establishes E-learning in Schools. New Era. https://neweralive.na/posts/ministry-of-education-establishes-e-learning-in-schools.

Sintema, E. J. (2020). "Effect of COVID 19 on the Performance of Grade 12 Students: Implications for STEM Education". *Eurasia Journal of Mathematics, Science and Technology Education*, 16(7). https://doi.org/10.29333/ejmste/7893.

Siririka, P. The Status of Education during and Post-Covid 19. New Era Publication. 2020-09-30 viewed 24 December 2022. https://neweralive.na/posts/the-status-of-education-during-and-post-Covid19.

The Namibian Constitution, Act 1 of 1990 as amended.

Thompson, A. (2013). "Exploring Radio, Convergence and Development in Africa". Nokoko, 3. Retrieved from https://ojs.library.carleton.ca/index.php/nokoko/issue/view/125.

UNESCO. (2012, November 28). 42 percent of African School Children Will Drop Out Before the End of Primary Education. Retrieved from http://www.unesco.org/new/en/member-states/single-view/news/42_of_african_school_children_will_drop_out_before_the_end/.

Unhale, S. S., Bilal, Q., Sanap, S., Thakhre, S., Wadatkar, S., Bairagi, R., Sagrule, S., & Biyani, K. (2020). "A Review on Corona Virus (COVID 19)". *International Journal of Pharmaceutical and Life Sciences*, 6(4), 109–115.

Wilhelm, J. P., & Lorgerie, P. (2020). #World Radio Day: Why Radio is Still Going Strong in Africa. Deuch Welle TV. Retrieved from https://www.dw.com/en/worldradioday-why-radio-is-still-going-strong-in-africa/a-52355828.

World Internet Users Statistics. (2020). World Internet Users and 2020 Population Stats. Retrieved from https://www.internetworldstats.com/stats.htm.

Yue, X.-G., Wang, C., Cheng, Z., & McAleer, M. (2020). "Risk Management of COVID 19 by Universities in China". *Journal of Risk and Financial Management*, 13(2). Retrieved from https://www.mdpi.com/1911-8074/13/2/36#.

Yuen, K., Ye, Z.-Wei, Fung, S., Chan, C., & Jin, D. (2020). "SARS-CoV-2 and COVID 19: The Most Important Research Questions". *Cell & Bioscience*. https://doi.org/10.1186/s13578-020-00404-4.

Zu, Z. Y., Jiang, M. D., Xu, P., Chen, W., Ni, Q., Lu, G. M., & Zhang, L. (2020). "Coronavirus Disease 2019 (COVID 19): A Perspective from China". *Radiography*, 294(2). https://doi.org/10.1148/radiol.2020200490.

Chapter 10

Bridging the Digital Divide in Education Sector amid COVID-19 Pandemic

Issues and Challenges in Tanzania

Abdallah Ally and Monika Ndapandula Shifotoka

INTRODUCTION

The coronavirus (COVID-19) pandemic is one of the infectious diseases that attracted broader attention in various international media and affected the lives of people vastly. Although COVID-19 is a health crisis, its impacts have gone beyond health crisis and threatened the social, economic, and political stability of various countries. The tourism industry is one of the sectors that was affected greatly due to restrictions that were imposed in various countries. As a result, most of the businesses shivered and workers were required to stay home (UNDP 2020, 15). Various fiscal measures were implemented to mitigate the adverse effect and provide relief for businesses and households. Irrespective of the variations in the effect of COVID-19 on the economies of nations, it is agreeable that COVID-19 unsympathetically affected the global economy. However, severe pressure will be noticed in most third-world countries due to poverty and weak and ineffective leadership.

The ineffective leadership and political instability in some African governments amplified COVID-19 as a threat to national security. The UN Security Council, in its Resolution 1308 (2000), acknowledged the potential of an epidemic to pose risk to stability and security and declared a "peaceful war against AIDS." In addition, after a SARS outbreak in 2003, a H1N1 pandemic in 2009, and an Ebola outbreak in 2014, which the UN Security Council Resolution 2177 marked as a "threat to international peace and security," more attention has been given to the concept of global health security (Rokvić & Jeftić 2015).

Although the mutual definition of health security is missing, the analysis of literature and several reports reveal that this concept is associated with the mass spread of infectious diseases, frightening not only individuals but society as a whole. The pathogen microorganisms can be used as biological weapons, which invokes military repercussions thereby endangering the stability and security of a country and region (Rokvić & Jeftić 2015). Regardless of the pandemic's effects on the socioeconomic and political stability of various nations worldwide, the focus of this chapter is mainly on its effects on children's rights and specifically access to education amid the COVID-19 pandemic.

CHILDREN'S RIGHTS AMID COVID-19

According to Human Rights Watch (2020), income loss and economic insecurity caused by lockdowns and other restrictions on freedom of movement have exposed children to social and economic threats. The increasing rate of deaths caused by the pandemic has caused a large number of children to be orphans and vulnerable to mistreatment. The worldwide economic depression caused by the COVID-19 crisis has jeopardized children's rights and exposed them to economic threats and social abuse. About 152 million children were already engaged in child labor before the COVID-19 pandemic, with a 73 million engaged in hazardous work (Human Rights Watch 2020). This is excerbated by the financial impotence of some families, family instability, and lack of peace, security, and justice, which have invited children into potential harm. (Human Rights Watch 2020, 6).

Government intervention is very important at this stage to rescue children entering the workforce and help their families survive. Each year, 12 million girls are married before reaching a legally accepted age for marriage. The economic hardships have influenced and are still influencing vulnerable families to espouse daughters off as soon as possible to reduce the number of people in the household to feed. Dowry and bride price practices sometimes mean that families in a financial crisis have a monetary incentive for arranging a marriage (Human Rights Watch 2020, 6).

IMPACTS OF COVID-19 ON EDUCATION

The effects of COVID-19 engulfed the education sector due to extended school closures (OECD 2020). Several countries announced school closures in March 2020 to mitigate the risks of the pandemic. During this time, varied measures and strategic plans were laid down to reconcile the situation.

Public and private institutions came up with online learning arrangements as a mitigation strategy. The idea behind this choice was to cover the gap caused by COVID-19. Most students who had a conducive learning environment adopted this system, referred to as homeschooling under the support of parental supervision. This arrangement kept the learners active and made teachers and schools responsible for the learning activities. In other countries, schools were partially open for parents working in essential sectors (OECD 2020, 3). However, this kind of arrangement excluded a good number of students due to internet accessibility, and financial and social limitations, causing great discrepancies among families.

Access to reliable internet services affected some students in both urban and rural areas and made them struggle with pains of the e-learning platform. For example, the OECD (2020) policy responses to COVID-19 revealed that 95 percent of students in Switzerland, Norway, and Austria were afforded computer facilities to use for their schoolwork, only 34 percent in Indonesia were. The same trend was also experienced in the US between privileged and disadvantaged families. The findings revealed that while about 25 percent of those from needy families had no access to a computer all. Regardless of the arrangements that were made for the provision of digital equipment to students from underprivileged families in New South Wales, Australia, there is a general concern that the pandemic has widened the digital divide (World Economic Forum 2020).

In Africa, the pandemic affected and held back the education system. It is estimated that about 200 million children and adolescents were not learning due to school closures. In the West and Central African regions, the nationwide closures of schools impacted about 140 million children (ADEA 2020). Urgent measures were instituted by governments and key education stakeholders to guarantee minimum interference in the teaching-learning process as schools were closed. The measures that were taken assured the continuity of education while the schools have been closed. Although the e-learning approach was expected to guarantee the learning process during the lockdown, many disadvantaged children were excluded due to internet challenges. In remote parts of Kenya, such as Kajiado, Narok, Samburu, Turkana, and Kilifi counties, electricity continued to be a stumbling block (Parsitau & Jepkemei 2020). Smartphones could have been an immediate solution for most rural dwellers; however, poverty and tensions around privacy and the cost of the internet were barriers (Parsitau & Jepkemei 2020).

In Tanzania, the effects of the pandemic were very clear in the education sector during the lockdown. The digital divide could be easily noticed among students and schools. E-learning platforms such as Google Classrooms were aggressively used by students coming from good-quality private schools, while the majority of students coming from disadvantaged families and those in public schools missed the opportunity. Although the government intervened in the situation to support the remote learning process, the challenges were on accessibility and affordability of internet and computer appliances among students.

DIGITAL TECHNOLOGY IN EDUCATION

The twenty-first century is considered an era of information and communication technologies (ICTs). ICT technology is playing a substantial role in our lives and is a base for economic growth and social developments. Most countries have achieved economic growth through ICT applications (Ma 2017, 2). The growth of this technology has been incorporated into the education industry and has become a vibrant component at all levels of education. The government's effort to promote the e-learning environment has grown significantly and has been incorporated into various official documents. The last fifteen years have experienced significant transformation in the education systems in most developed and developing countries through the incorporation of ICT in the learning system (OECD 2016).

Detailed educational ICT strategies grounded around the broad aim of inspiring and supporting schools' use of computers, the internet, and other digital technologies have been documented in all developed countries. These strategies involve devoting substantial amounts of funding towards computer hardware and internet connectivity to ensure internet accessibility for pupils and teachers. Training of teachers and adjustments of curricula to include technology use forms part of the strategies. In Ethiopia and Estonia, for example (ICT in Education Implementation Strategy) digital technology forms a central part in modernizing the education systems (Selwyn 2011, 36). Countries like China, Taiwan, South Korea, and Singapore have a set of policies geared toward the promotion of e-literacy and digital skills in secondary and tertiary education. Although there is a growing promise to increase e-literacy in less developing nations, the shortage of e-learning facilities and the disparity in the access and use of technology hamper the process (ICT) (Ma 2017).

Tanzania decided to provide a national framework to enable ICT to contribute to achieving national development goals and transform Tanzania into a knowledge-based society in its first national ICT policy of 2003 (Kafyulilo 2010, 16). Though the 2003 policy mentioned education as one of the areas of its focus, the policy was too vague and did not state specific components of ICT integration in education. In 2007, the ICT policy for basic education was framed, aiming at promoting the acquisition of knowledge, skills, and understanding for the development and improvement of man and society

(Kafyulilo 2010). The policy provided room for ICT application from pre-primary to teacher education and wide use of technology in non-formal and adult education. The policy aimed to lead the incorporation of ICT in basic education. The policy provided for a variety of technologies, including radio, mobile telephony, computers, and the internet. It aimed at empowering learners, teachers, education managers, and leaders to use ICT prudently and efficiently for expanding learning opportunities. Even though there are signs of rapid progress in ICT infrastructure in Tanzania, communication facilities are still dominant in urban areas, leaving the rural areas underserved (Kafyulilo 2010).

The internet penetration in Tanzania reached 43 percent in 2018, with 48.77 percent of the mobile phone subscribers using the internet (TCRA 2019). While other sectors, such as banking, are taking advantage of this technology, the education sector has not been aggressive enough in using this technology to deliver services to rural communities. The e-learning services are more dominant in private schools as compared to government schools. According to the Global e-Schools and Communities Initiative (2010) education analysis report, about half of the public-registered secondary schools in Tanzania are in rural areas with poor communication setup. The existing gap in internet connectivity and access to e-learning services between advantaged and disadvantaged groups and among schools is leading to disparities in educational success.

THE DIGITAL DIVIDE

The digital divide is a term that refers to the gap between demographics and regions that have access to modern information and communications technology and those that do not have access. These technologies are smartphones, television, personal computers, and the internet. Despite the developments made in technology, poverty, poor infrastructure, corruption, and bureaucracy and political will have widened the digital gap (Ma 2012). Ma (2012) reveals that deliberate efforts of policymakers, educators, and entrepreneurs in developed countries have greatly contributed to the decline in the digital divide. However, the situation is different in less-developed countries, where the gap between the socioeconomically advantaged and the disadvantaged is larger.

The eruption of COVID-19 in both developed and developing countries caused millions of children to be affected by school closures aimed at slowing the transmission of the pandemic. To accommodate the situation, various strategies were implemented to allow the learning process to occur. Various e-learning platforms were developed, including the provision of education through radio and television and the distribution of printed learning materials, among other options. All these strategies were aimed at mitigating the negative effects of COVID-19 and ensuring that learning is not interrupted (UNICEF 2020).

Although the strategies had a positive purpose, their fruits failed to capture children coming from vulnerable families (UNICEF 2020, 1). In Tanzania, for example, a month after the announcement of the first COVID-19 case in the country, the government urged parents to ensure that they optimally utilize the virtual learning opportunity. Several learning arrangements were proposed and implemented; however, the arrangements were useful to a small segment of the population. Tanzania Institute of Education created an online platform where online textbooks from pre-primary to advanced secondary education could be accessed. This option applied to a small segment of the population whose families were able to support internet facilities and have the required facilities to access the online learning content. In general, the option was utilized by a small segment of the population, as the majority of students in Tanzania could not access the internet at home due to internet accessibility, lack of ICT accessories, and broadband costs (Todd 2020).

Other options that were also implemented to support learning during the COVID-19 pandemic included learning through TV and radio broadcasts. These options could not reach and help all students due to a lack of access to essential facilities. According to the Household Budget Survey (2017–2018), only 43 percent of the households had TV sets, 24 percent had radio sets, and 78 percent had mobile phones. This means not all families, especially the poor ones, could support their children in learning through these channels. The use of information technology was a powerful tool to mitigate the challenges of COVID-19; however, many of the Tanzania population could not afford the costs of such technologies. According to the Tanzania Communication Regulatory Authority (TCRA) report of December 2019, Tanzania had 25.7 million internet users. The average cost of internet use is still high; the cost of 75 MBs, which could hardly be enough per child per day, was Tsh.1,000, which is Tsh.30,000 per month. This cost can be afforded by very few families.

THE RIGHT TO EDUCATION IN DIGITAL AGE

Technology in education provides important benefits, but it can also impair the right to education. While a digital device-based education can bring advantages in the form of access to a computer or electronic device, when students or schools lack the financial means to obtain access, they fall behind. When only some schools are provided with technology or when private schools can afford better technology, existing social divisions in education outcomes will increase. In this respect, governments are compelled under international law to provide resources for the realization of the right to education (United Nations 2016). In recognition and protection of Internet Rights, Article 1 of the African declaration provides that:

> The fundamental rights of every individual enshrined in the Universal Declaration of Human Rights of the United Nations, the Charter of Fundamental Rights of the European Union, national constitutions, and other relevant international declarations shall be protected on the Internet.

Under Article 3 (4), public institutions are required to promote, especially through the educational and training system, the informed use of the internet and should take steps to eliminate any form of cultural lag that might preclude or limit the use of the internet by any person. In realization of this, governments are required to dedicate a reasonable budget to education and ensure that a legal framework that provides for sustainable political and financial support is in place. Besides, the application of ICT in education should conform to the standards stipulated by international instruments. It is important to ensure that the principles and norms of the right to education are preserved when using information and communications technologies (United Nations 2016).

The right to education has been given room in Tanzanian laws, including the Constitution, as a fundamental objective and directive principle of state policy. Article 11(2) of the Constitution of the United Republic of Tanzania warranties this right to all citizens up to the highest level according to their merits and abilities. The weakness of this provision is that it is not a basic right. Being just a constitutional right falling outside the provisions of fundamental rights jeopardizes its enforceability under the Basic Rights and Duties Enforcement Act (Act no. 33 of 1994). The right to education is recognized by various international instruments. Article 26 of the Universal Declaration of Human Rights, Article 13 of the International Covenant on Economic, Social and Cultural Rights (ICESCR), and Article 28 of the Convention on the Rights of the Child (CRC) lay down similar rights. The Convention against Discrimination in Education, 1960, directs governments to formulate, develop, and apply national policies that will promote equality in education. The motive behind all these directives is to ensure equality as well as equity (UNESCO 2020).

These provisions have been very useful in the decision of various cases in courts. In the case of *Timishev v. Russia* No. 55762/00 and 55974/00, the court considered unequal treatment to constitute discrimination. In the case of *Yean and Bosico v. the Dominican Republic* (2005), in consideration of the same arguments, the court stated that the state must provide free primary education to all children in an appropriate environment and in the conditions necessary to ensure their full intellectual development. The African Commission on Human and Peoples' Rights went further in the interpretation by considering the mismanagement of public finances and the closure of universities and secondary schools for two years as a violation of the African Charter in the case of Free Legal Assistance Group and others vs. Zaire, Comm. No. 25/89, 47/90, 56/91, 100/93 (1995).

BRIDGING THE DIGITAL DIVIDE

Alleviating information and technology disparities amongst populations is amazingly important. To fill the gaps and address the ICT disparities, effective and reasonably priced ICT infrastructure combined with enabling legal environments are vital. Various governments in the world have taken several initiatives to address the challenges of the digital divide. The Indian government, for example, has a Digital India Campaign to increase internet connectivity and make the country empowered in the field of technology. The Community Technology Center's program and The Neighborhood Networks Program have been created by the US government (Grasmick 2015).

To eliminate the digital divide in Illinois, the Illinois General Assembly enacted the "Eliminate the Digital Divide" law to create a fund to help develop information technology infrastructure by purchasing IT goods and services (Grasmick 2015). Other countries have included access to the internet as a fundamental right in the relevant legal systems. Estonia, Greece, and Ecuador have included the right in the constitution, while Finland and Peru have it by law. The existence of the right to education in France and Costa Rica is obtained in some cases by the laws of the respective domestic courts (Frosini 2014, 5–12). The recognition of digital knowledge and the efforts to bridge the digital divide are heavily emphasized in the 2030 Agenda for Sustainable Development (United Nations 2016). The development of the tailored programs and infrastructure to allow internet access and enhance the regulatory and market environment is pioneered by ITU in all regions (ITU 2019).

The government of Tanzania has taken initiatives to ensure that communication as a universal right is accessible to its entire population. The Universal Communications Service Access Fund (UCSAF) was established under the Universal Communications Service Access Act, Cap 422, which was assented to by the President of the United Republic of Tanzania in January 2007. Although the fund is aimed at reducing the digital divide, its achievement is not well recognized.

POST-COVID-19 IMPACTS AND ITS IMPLICATIONS IN EDUCATION SECTOR

The COVID-19 pandemic has taught the world and visibly disclosed all the existing gaps, weaknesses, and challenges people are facing in both developed and developing nations. Although COVID-19 is no longer dominating the news, it is still roaming around, and there are new cases and the possibility of new waves (UN 2022). It has weakened and affected seriously the global economy and raised havoc and fear in the social, health, and education sectors. It is estimated that the COVID-19 impacts might push about 60 million people into extreme poverty worldwide, with 27 million people living in sub-Saharan African countries such as Tanzania (Shao et al., 2022). In response to the economic crisis caused by the pandemic, central banks across developed and developing countries have put in place mitigation strategies to overcome the crisis by slashing interest rates, injecting liquidity, and providing emergency funding for firms and households (Kumar 2020).

In the education sector, the post-COVID-19 challenges have pushed schools and colleges to adopt digital technologies and make alterations in the management and administration of education services. Several universities across Africa, including ones in countries such as Egypt, Ghana, South Africa, and Rwanda, have transformed some of their courses to online platforms during and after the COVID-19 pandemic (TCU 2022). In Tanzania, higher learning institutions have also adopted technology-enhanced teaching and learning during and after COVID-19. The adoption has assisted the growth of online teachings through ZOOM-technology and MOODLE (Mtebe et al., 2021).

In strengthening the transformation, in the year 2022, the Commission for Universities in Tanzania (TCU) issued Guidelines for Online and Blended Delivery Modes of Courses for University Institutions in Tanzania to address post-COVID-19 challenges. In addition to that, universities have expressed interest to develop programs that can either be offered fully online or in a mixed mode with traditional face-to-face systems. However, while the education system is going online in some courses, the transformation has not bridged the existing social disparities that have caused a good segment of people to be marginalized from the platform. E-learning has not been friendly to the majority of the population due to constraining technology inclusion factors (Zgovu 2021). It is the opinion of various stakeholders that the transformation should go hand in hand with the government efforts in improving pedagogical skills for secondary and primary teachers and upgrading telecommunication infrastructure to augment internet affordability and accessibility to all people. Before the COVID-19 crisis, the Tanzania government was working toward improving the digital infrastructure in the country and the capacity of teachers in that regard. The training is part of the implementation of the National ICT

Policy of 2003, which was revised in 2016, and the Education and Training Policy of 2014. Both policies inspire the use of ICT in the teaching and learning process at various levels of education (ILO 2021).

However, as schools and universities are going online, there are still some policy and legal gaps in the adoption of e-learning. The existing regulatory and policy framework does not effectively answer the digital technology challenges and offer a solution to bridging the digital divide. While many developed countries have specific e-learning policies, frameworks, regulations, and funding bodies, these are not available in developing countries. The Partnership for Higher Education in Africa's (PHEA) e-Learning Initiative does not have specific national policies devoted to e-learning, although education is mentioned in national ICT policies. The PHEA countries are Egypt, Ghana, Kenya, Madagascar, Mozambique, Nigeria, South Africa, Tanzania, and Uganda (Bryan 2018).

CONCLUSION

Nearly half of Tanzania's population is not benefiting from the current digital economy due to internet connectivity. A study carried out by RIA (2017) reported that 86 percent of the rural population remains unconnected to internet services. This situation does not align with the Tanzania National Development Vision 2025, which envisions transforming this nation into a middle-income country. The vision aims in establishing a knowledgeable and learning society that enjoys a high quality of livelihood. It also emphasizes promoting science and technology in education as among the core values of the document. Although the paper guarantees such transformations, the realities on the ground do not tally and match with the vision. Most public secondary schools in rural and urban areas do not have essential facilities to support the proper exploitation of ICT in the education industry. Although ICT has been incorporated in primary and secondary school curricula, it appears to be mere cosmetic than reality, as there are not enough facilities to utilize the technology (Nyirenda 2013). To achieve digital inclusion strategies, the right to education should be given the status of a basic right in the constitution to make it enforceable under the *Basic Rights* and *Duties Enforcement Act* 1994 (Act no 33 of 1994).

REFERENCES

Association for the Development of Education in Africa (ADEA). Delivering Education at Home in African Member States Amid the Covid 19 Pandemic: Country Status Report (2020).

Bryan, Lugemwa. E-learning Policies and E-learning Acceptance and Usage, Operations Research Society of Eastern Africa (ORSEA) Journal, 2018.

Grasmick, Brittany. Recognizing "Access to Information" as a Basic Human Right: A Necessary Step in Enforcing Human Rights Provisions within Free Trade Agreements, Loyola University. *Chicago International Law Review*, 12(2), 2015, 214–230.

Human Rights Watch, COVID 19 and Children's Rights, 2020.

Kagoya, Sumaya M. The Use of Digital Transformation to Address Education Challenges Caused by COVID 19 in Developing Countries. *Social Sciences*, 9(6), 2020, 233–240.

Kuo-Hsun, Ma. The Inequality of Digital Learning among Students in Rich and Poor Countries. Doctoral Dissertations, University of Connecticut, 2017.

Mishra, Mukesh Kumar. The World after COVID 19 and its Impact on Global Economy, ZBW – Leibniz Information Centre for Economics, Kiel, Hamburg, 2020.

Mtebe, Joel S., Fulgence, Katherine, and Galagher, Michael. COVID 19 and Technology Enhanced Teaching in Higher Education in Sub-Saharan Africa: A Case of the University of Dar es Salaam, Tanzania. *Journal of Learning for Development, JL4D*, 8(2), 2021, 383–397.

Mtebe, Joel, and Gallagher, Michael. Continued Usage Intentions of Digital Technologies Post-Pandemic through the Expectation-Confirmation Model: The Case of a Tanzanian University. *International Journal of Education and Development using Information and Communication Technology (IJEDICT)*, 18(1), 2022, 125–145.

Mwakyusa, Wilson Pholld, and Ng`webeya, Lucas Masome. (2022). The Response of Tanzania Higher Learning Institutions to E- Learning during Covid 19 Pandemic. *East African Journal of Education and Social Sciences*, 3(1), 2022, 19–28. https://doi.org/10.46606/eajess2022v03i01.0142

Nyirenda, Masozi. Planning for ICT Literacy in Public Schools in Tanzania, 2013. Available at https;?www.ifg.cc/aktuelles/nachrichten/regionen/284-tz-tansania-tanzania/45453-planning-for-ict-literacy-in-public-schools-in-tanzania

OECD. Access to Justice and the COVID 19 Pandemic, Compendium of Country Practices, 2020.

OECD. Innovating Education and Educating for Innovation, the Power of Digital Technologies and Skills, OECD Publishing, Paris, 2016.

OECD. Supporting the Continuation of Teaching and Learning during the COVID 19 Pandemic, 2020.

Parsitau, Damaris Seleina, and Jepkemei, Evelyn. How School Closure during COVID 19 Further Marginalize Vulnerable Children in Kenya, 2020.

TCU. Guidelines for Online and Blended Delivery Modes of Courses for University Institutions in Tanzania, 2022.

Todd, Gemma. COVID 19 and Education Systems in Tanzania: Brainstorming for a True Ed-tech Disruption?, 2020.

Trade Union Advisory Committee to the OECD. Impact and Implications of the COVID 19-Crisis on Educational Systems and Households, 2020.

UN. Impact of the PANDEMIC on Trade and Development, Lessons Learned, 2022.

UNDP. Rapid Socio-Economic Impact Assessment of COVI-19 in Tanzania, 2020.

UNESCO. Education in a Post-COVID World: Nine Ideas for Public Action International Commission on the Futures of Education, 2020.
UNESCO. The Right to Education for All: Ten Reasons Why the Convention against Discrimination in Education is Highly Significant in Today's World, 2007. https://unesdoc.unesco.org/ark:/48223/pf0000153765
UNESCO. Why the Convention against Discrimination in Education is Highly Significant in Today's World, The Convention against Discrimination in Education, 2005 (1960).
United Nations. Report of the Special Rapporteur on the Right to Education, 2016.
Vanja, Rokvić and Jeftić, Zoran. Health Issues as Security Issues. *Vojno delo*, 67, br. 6, str. 2015, 53–69.
Zgovu, Evious K. Technology as an Enabler for Addressing the COVID 19 Challenges in the East African Community. AERC Working Paper – COVID 19_021 African Economic Research Consortium, Nairobi, 2021.

Conclusion

Reflections on Salient Lessons Learned

Masake Pilisano Harris and
Iroanya Obinna Richard

The COVID-19 pandemic exposed the weaknesses inherent in the social infrastructure of African states, especially healthcare and social security systems. African states were characterized by a high level of unpreparedness and scientific and technological insufficiency. These, in turn, worsened the impact of COVID-19 on all fronts; thus, high mortality rate, rampant job losses, and arbitrary and erratic state responses were experienced in most African states. If anything, the pandemic revealed that in times of global disasters, the preoccupation of states is national security and survival at the expense of globalization or collective security. This entails that the essence of collective international effort, or the so-called march toward a "global village" is more theoretical than real. The abstract construct was tested by the global pandemic and proved unsustainable in practice in times of crises.

The effect of preferring national security and survival over collective international effort in times of global pandemic is strongly felt in poor and developing states owing to the weakness of their economies. While developed countries were not spared by COVID-19 pandemic, the relative strength of their economies, scientific knowledge and skills, and technological and industrial capacities enabled them to develop life-saving vaccines whose administration and distribution were initially prioritized and limited to nationals and citizens first. Inevitably, such actions raised suspicions and allegations of vaccine apartheid against developed states by developing states.

The wrath of the pandemic begged for more questions on security and the survival of the poor and developing (less industrialized) states. Besides high mortalities, COVID-19 pandemic weakened fragile public health systems and stressed economies to the brink of collapse across Africa. The measures taken by sovereign states in Africa seemed not to have taken into consideration the short-term and long-term effects of the pandemic. Instead, these measures limited fundamental human rights, particularly the right to fair trial, association, assembly, movement, and the press.

Curiously, these measures exposed gaps in sociopolitical protection of immigrants, the undocumented, and refugees in host nations. Gleaned from these patent errors in the choice of security strategies adopted by states, there are important lessons that may be noted. To effectively mitigate future pandemics, the states need to rise above national interests. This has the potential to collectively empower and complement each other in the fight against the pandemic. The call for collective global efforts during global pandemic is distinguishable from strategies often adopted to address aggressive wars, where states may face a non-alignment dilemma that riddles Africa.

Domestically, states of emergency were declared. These declarations were, however, paradoxical. Though targeted at subduing the pandemic, it ended up opening the floodgates of arbitrary and unethical conduct by the executive organs of states. Most visible was the use of force. The executive organs of state's counterpandemic regulations were hurriedly drafted and were an affront to the Bill of Rights. These repugnant regulations were enforced stringently, leading to police and military brutality against societies that were already victimized by COVID-19. Critical to these arbitrary uses of power by the executive was the issue of lack of responsive legislative framework capable of countering health pandemic. This left the executive organs of states to pass decrees or regulations that regulated social and health issues. It is prudent, as a lesson learned from the COVID-19 pandemic, that responsive and resilient legislative frameworks capable of withstanding pandemic's legal shortfalls be adopted.

The lack of a responsive legal framework created confusion over the question of vaccination. There were a mix of approaches to the question of vaccination: voluntary or mandatory. In some states, vaccination was made a prerequisite to access to several services, such as travel (domestic or international), and workplaces, and so on. These disguised mandatory vaccination tactics were applied inconsistently because of the lack of legislative clarity on the issue.

The mainstream and alternative dispute resolution mechanisms were not spared by the effects of the COVID-19 pandemic. The justice system is a critical component of social cohesion in African states, particularly in conflict-ridden states. It is not in doubt that COVID-19 exacerbated a backlog of court cases, leading to the question of delayed delivery of justice because the courts were closed. In addition, peace negotiations in conflict-prone countries were on the brink of collapse. Circumventing these challenges, particularly in the judiciary, required the convergence of technology and the justice systems.

The judiciary should therefore invest in technology to ensure that courts can be held virtually without being limited to the traditional practice of in-person approach.

The COVID-19 pandemic raised tensions and widened the gap between state and society, the rich and poor. African states are inexplicably inhabited by poverty-stricken majority who live in densely populated informal settlements, squalors, and deprived villages with no access to clean water, sanitation facilities, or a tracing system. These factors rendered it difficult to contain the COVID-19 pandemic optimally in informal settlements across the continent. The aspiration to resolve these challenges hinged on budgetary constraints and political will. The impact of COVID-19 on poverty-stricken informal settlements should be used to inform policy direction, urban planning, and land use in preparation for the future.

Pandemic control measures raised serious ethical, behavioral, and leadership questions necessitating the call for the inculcation, from a young age, of ethical values in African populations. The endemic problem of corruption, which has been the bane of African societies, manifested prominently during the pandemic outbreak. Reported cases of COVID-19 violations by state officials and discrepancies in the distribution of palliatives to less privileged populations highlighted the need to effectively address this problem through reconscientization programs. There is a need to call for the strengthening of judicial systems across Africa, and the criminal justice system should play a crucial role during periods of global pandemic outbreaks alongside the police to provide effective leadership.

While in reality one cannot completely avoid disparity between developed and less developed states or the privileging of lives in the developed world over lives in the less developed world in the age of globalization and digitization, ethics demands fair treatment of all. Polarization of societies along ethnicity and socioeconomic status as manifested in differential living quarters for the wealthy and politically connected and the low socioeconomic status influenced the extent of COVID-19 regulation and enforcement.

In the living quarters of low socioeconomic groups, police brutality and gross human rights abuses were a daily occurrence. Unethical, selective brutality by the police and military did not achieve the goal of preventing or limiting the spread of the virus. The rate of infection was high among low socioeconomic groups who were cramped in small living spaces and could not observe social distancing and isolation at home but were forced to stay indoors by the authorities.

Cruel, degrading, and inhumane punishment exacerbated the failure of states to objectively investigate and prosecute alleged violations. This argument does not disregard or downplay the contributions of the armed forces and the police in protecting sovereignty and territorial integrity of African states and ensuring public safety and security during COVID-19. The crust of the argument is that positive contributions made by the security cluster agencies during COVID-19 outbreak in different parts of Africa became overshadowed by gross human rights abuses. A critical concern regarding the use of the military internally was obvious, necessitated by the lack of preparedness. States will continue to use the military in complementary roles in Africa. However, such deployments have to be done without compromising military professionalism. Lessons learned from COVID-19 should inform future policies in this regard at the strategic level. Operationally, domestic deployment of military forces must adopt some components of the Fused Security Era.

The devastating effects of COVID-19 raged globally but never compelled collective global efforts needed to fight it and protect humanity. Thus, security sector governance, differential legal and sociocultural systems, and the availability of resources meant that enforcement of COVID-19 regulations varied. Essentially, the readiness of security cluster agencies to tackle the challenge of global pandemic came under intense scrutiny of citizens. A critical revelation was that African states have not done enough in terms of improving the living conditions of people, which had a reverberating effect on efforts to control and manage domestic health crises such as COVID-19.

In reality, efforts aimed at containing the spread of COVID-19 in different African states were hampered by countless socioeconomic challenges, for example, poverty, unemployment, and a lack of or poor social safety nets. These social conditions contributed to non-compliance with the state of emergency regulations to a significant extent. Besides the government's approach, the public sector's governance complicated the whole aspect of managing public health. For instance, poor housing, water scarcity, and poor infrastructure undermined the security sector's capacity to mitigate the deadly COVID-19.

The COVID-19 pandemic revealed policy and infrastructural deficits of African states, especially in the health sector. But most importantly, it also threw into limelight the mistreatment of African migrants in Africa. Interestingly, while global COVID-19 vaccine nationalism limited access to vaccines for African states, lack of proper documentation prevented migrants from accessing healthcare services in host countries. Evidence has shown that integrating migrants into host economies can assist in local capacity development. However, COVID-19 pandemic showed how anemic the policy landscape is when it comes to migration. The undocumented population was disenfranchised from accessing health services as well as regarded as a threat to national security. The costs of exclusionary policies have become glaring in the era of COVID-19 and have led to the displacement of some survival immigrants and the unfortunate return of others to the situations that they were fleeing from in their home countries. COVID-19 restrictions affected the economic and social well-being of refugees. This marginalized group was, in addition, isolated and excluded from palliative measures launched by governments to provide basic food supplies to vulnerable populations.

Although COVID-19 pandemic may have ended, as the WHO has declared, there are still post-pandemic challenges confronting African states. Adjusting to the post-pandemic era would require reviving and strengthening economies to create employment for citizens, improving social infrastructure, and relooking into legal systems to plug loopholes identified during the pandemic. The questions that come to the fore include: are we out of the woods with the COVID-19 pandemic? Is a complete transition from COVID-19 era to post-COVID-19 era possible? What can we expect in the post-COVID-19 era?

Addressing these questions requires delving into the history of pandemics. Historically, the 21st century, notwithstanding increased scientific knowledge, has witnessed the rise of pandemics to a point that full clearance out of the woods on pandemics is not possible to predict. Predictively, based on the patterns and incursions of global pandemics, it appears that pandemics are bound to occur in future. This presupposition is premised on the observed patterns so far; for instance, in 1918–1919 the spread of influenza pandemic reportedly claimed over 50 million deaths. In 1957–1958, an influenza (H2N2) pandemic outbreak was detected in East Asia. Shortly thereafter, in 1968, another influenza (H3N2) sagged and claimed thousands of lives. In 2002, the severe acute respiratory syndrome (SARS) outbreak was detected in China that claimed about 800 deaths. The 2009 influenza pandemic outbreak (H1N1) claimed over 200 000 deaths. In 2012, the Middle East Respiratory Syndrome (MERS-COV) was detected. In 2019, the COVID-19 pandemic outbreak with a high mortality rate was detected. There were other health pandemics such as HIV/AIDS outbreak worldwide in the 1980s and the 1976 Ebola pandemic outbreak. To date, about 24 Ebola outbreaks have since been detected in Africa, of which the 2013–2016 period saw the largest outbreak that claimed about 12,000 deaths.

The frequency of the occurrence of these pandemics does not preclude the incursion of pandemics in the near future. However, with the WHO pronouncement that COVID-19 is no longer a global health pandemic, this signifies the transitory path to post COVID-19 era. In essence, this does not necessarily imply that COVID-19 is eradicated; rather, there could still be COVID-19 cases reported. In addition, this could entail availability of vaccine, and other mitigation measures that ease the effects of the pandemic. In a nutshell, it is arguable that nations have reached the post-COVID-19 era. The post-COVID-19 era raises further questions, among others: What should society expect? There are several issues, from a social, legal, and ethical perspective, that may be prevalent and expected in the post-COVID-19 era. These include trends in labor, human security, dependency, and uncertainties regarding finance, economic structure, human cost, and education.

Labor issues: Labor forms part of a broader social issue in any given society. As elucidated above, COVID-19 negatively impacted the labor industry. Employees and workers were laid off, businesses were closed, and migrated and adopted new methods of labor practice, such as working from home (remote work). To this extent, there are several labor issues that are expected in the post-COVID-19 era, among them growth of the remote work—business entities, especially, large corporations, during COVID-19, invested in technology to afford them to operate remotely. The adoption of remote work policies and infrastructure will persist in the post-COVID-19 era. However, remote work influences changes to other factors, that is, digitalization and revision of skill sets that may be required for hiring purposes. These skills include use of technology and ICT. It is paramount that employees need to reskill and relearn new skills or risk to be laid off under the redundancy rules. The consequences, therefore, place more pressure on employees to scale up and increase business costs due to investment in technology, digitization, cybersecurity, and staff training. A long-term benefit of the adoption and incorporation of remote work policies, infrastructure, and employee reskilling is to build a robust and resilient capacity to be able to deal with any pandemic that may arise in the future. The level of preparedness in anticipation for any future pandemic outbreak will not be similar to the COVID-19 pandemic's lived experiences.

Human security: In the mix of any pandemic, there is a question of human security. Human security is a derivative concept that includes facets such as economic, food, health, environment, personal, community, and political dimensions. In the post-COVID-19 era, the expectation include that people will return to their normal ways of life, no curfews, no social distancing, or wearing of masks, and return to in person working environment. However, these human security dimensions are at risk and remain vulnerable, in most of the African states, to incursion of any future pandemic. This is because most African countries, in post-COVID-19 era, do not have facilities, right equipment, and technology to produce their own pharmaceutical products, i.e., vaccines to counter future pandemics. Further, there is lack of economic stability due to high levels of corruption and civil wars that are perennial, and the question of half-mast democracies.

Human cost: In the post-COVID-19 era, the question of human cost arises. Closely looking at the past pandemics, including COVID-19, it would appear that the devastating effects thereof include loss of lives, much so, children under the age of 5 and elderly persons above 50 years. The implications for human geography include irreplaceability of the lost lives and the creation of a bubble or gap, especially the deaths of children. This demographical consequence or gap will persist in the long term, robbing the nation's future of potentially active, effective, and productive economic and social players. At this juncture, it is important to signpost the zero-carbon argument. Unsupported security perceptions inked COVID-19 to be a weaponized biological pathogen with the objective of achieving a zero-carbon footprint. This argument, even though it is unsupported (as there is no evidence to these claims, yet), shows that, at a parallel level, the continued loss of children due to pandemics is problematic and it has the potential to negatively alter and affect the human demography and geography.

Acceleration of dependency: COVID-19 pandemic worsened the economic situation in most of the African states; it lowered the already fragile levels of gross domestic product per capita, reduced foreign direct investment, ostracized the marginalized and poor, increased inability to overcome economic crises, and raised the commodity prices to an all-time high. Most African states depleted their fiscus and reserves during the COVID-19 pandemic era. The implications, in the post-COVID-19 era, include that most African states would increasingly depend on aid, donations, and handouts that are seemingly from Asia, Russia, and global north and west. The dependency syndrome is not short of neocolonial tactic, as the former colonial powers would be scrambling for Africa for the provision of aid and handouts, which has the potential to exacerbate lack of innovation and deepen the poverty gullies in Africa.

Education: During the pandemic, educational institutions were forced to close and migrate from traditional methods of teaching and learning and adopt online methods. This transition proved difficult since most of the African states lacked the necessary infrastructure to effectively deliver online teaching, ranging from poor network coverage, lack of computers, lack of resources, technology apathy, and illiteracy in computing. Learners and teachers had to start utilizing online tools due to social distancing and closure of schools, resulting in a disparity in the provision of education. Lack of infrastructure, access, digital divide, and cyberattacks are some of the key challenges that the education system faced during the closure of schools. Those from disadvantaged and poor backgrounds were not able to learn during this period, so they lagged when the classes resumed.

The effect of COVID-19 was felt in the national examination results and beyond, and it has a long-term implications for the education system in Africa and globally. The impact might continue in the post-COVID-19 era, as there is no clear policy indication on how to deal with students who lagged due to the pandemic. When school resumed, the students who lagged had no choice but to repeat the grades or be promoted to the next grade without sufficiently demonstrating the requisite competencies. This has a long-term impact that goes beyond the remits of quality of education to economics and epistemological consequences.

With these lived realities, post-COVID-19 era has witnessed tremendous adjustments. Developing countries started exploring new ways of expanding information infrastructure and increasing access to ICTs by reducing the cost of service, especially when it comes to access to computers and internet. Governments have adopted various ICT and educational policies that are inclusive, taking the needs of learners from poor backgrounds into account. For instance, the implementation of hybrid methods of teaching and learning, promoting digital literacy, investing in ICT, internet, and digitalization. Further increased cooperation between private and public sectors, education, and the IT industry to provide cost-effective and affordable services for people.

There are uncertainties and potential threats that beset the post-COVID-19 era. These include reorganizing unbalanced budgeting and accountability. During COVID-19 pandemic, the bulk of the state budget was appropriated to boost and prioritize health over and above other social issues, such as the fight against corruption, etc. Post-COVID-19 pandemic studies reveal that procurement corruption was prevalent during COVID-19 era. This is partly because the ministries of health and other functionaries were exempted from following regular procurement checks and balances under the various state of emergency laws. The exemptions were abused, and consequently, there was proliferation of corruption and lack of accountability. Therefore, these eventualities have the potential to influence shortfalls in revenue, increases expenditure, and indebtedness.

Unemployment is a typical consequence that may ensue in the post-COVID-19 era. African states depleted their reserves while battling the pandemic, and even went further to borrow beyond their capacity for loan restructuring and payment. The implication that besets this indebtedness is that governments and private sector may not be able to generate adequate employment opportunities to absorb the growing number of unemployed, especially qualified youth. This is treacherous and may lead to severe social unrest through youth movements, boycotts, and demonstrations that may be disruptive.

Geopolitics and rivalry: COVID-19 unmasks true realities as to which state may be a foe or ally. The allies shared stringent resources including the vaccines, technologies, and so on, to intensify the fight against the pandemic. In contrast, some lines were drawn among states by prioritizing their nationals and even cutting on regular aid. The effects of reduced aid was much experienced in developing states—to the extent that vaccine apartheid was mooted. The impact of these consequences includes that the post-COVID-19 era would experience and signify the beginning of the end of the non-alignment era, which was adopted by many of the African states in their international relationships.

Index

About the Editors

Dr. Masake Pilisano Harris is an international law scholar with interest in legal, forensic, security, sociology, and international relations studies. He has enrolled as MBA candidate at NUST. He holds the following degrees: Doctor of Philosophy in Criminal Justice (UNISA), South Africa; LLD-public law: international criminal law (Stellenbosch University); LLM (Stellenbosch University); Masters in Policing Practice (Southern Business School); LLB and B-Juris (UNAM); Postgraduate Diploma in Procurement Management (NUST); and Postgraduate Certificate in Higher Education (NUST). Harris is a senior lecturer and associate dean for the School of Human Sciences and Education, Faculty of Commerce, Human Sciences and Education at the Namibia University of Science and Technology, Namibia. He was a former police officer with the rank of Detective Chief Inspector in the Namibian Police Force. He was also guest lecturer at Interpol School of Excellence in Harare, Zimbabwe, and at Police College, Namibia. He was former head of Secretariat (Namibian delegation) for the Sub-Committee to the Joint Security Commission between Namibia, Botswana, Zimbabwe, Zambia, and Angola (2003–2006). He was the co-founder of the *Unam Law Review* and served as Head Articles Editor until 2013. He is co-author of various articles and book chapters, including the book *The Law of Pre-Trial Criminal Procedure in Namibia*. He has also been serving in community engagement with the Namibia Red Cross Society, a nonprofit humanitarian-based institution. In addition, he's serving as a Listed Professional Investigator for the International Criminal Court (ICC). Harris is Admitted Legal Practitioner of High Court of Namibia and postdoc fellow of the Alexander von Humboldt Foundation at Humboldt University, Berlin, Germany.

Dr. Iroanya Obinna Richard holds a PhD in International Relations from the University of Pretoria. He is the immediate past associate dean of the School of Military Science at the University of Namibia, Windhoek, where he teaches Security and Strategic Studies. He was a recipient of the European Union Erasmus Mundus Scholarship in 2008 and the author of the book *Human Trafficking and Security in Southern Africa: The South African and Mozambican Experience* (2018). He is a co-editor of the book *Towards Africa-oriented Risk Analysis Models: A Contextual and Methodological Approach* (2008). In 2015, he was a guest lecturer at the South African National Defence College (SANDC) on its Security and Defence Studies Programme (SDSP) 01/15 and served as a postdoctoral research fellow at the Thabo Mbeki African Leadership Institute (TMALI), University of South Africa (UNISA), between 2015 and 2017. Before joining the University of Namibia, Richard Iroanya was a Research Fellow in the Department of Political Studies and International Relations at North-West University, Vaal Triangle Campus, in South Africa. His successful academic career has seen him work as a Senior Research Specialist at the Africa Institute of South Africa (AISA) in Pretoria (AISA is now a unit of the Human Sciences Research Council, HSRC) between 2004 and 2007. He is a scholar with in-depth empirical knowledge of community engagement and issues pertaining to peace and security and conflict transformation. He is quite knowledgeable about Africa's security dilemma and has experience in mentorship of young academics, teaching, research, planning, organization, implementation, and management of programs. Richard Iroanya has published extensively on issues of peace and security in Africa in forms of book chapters and journal articles.

About the Contributors

Dr. Abdallah Ally is a lecturer in the Faculty of Law at the Open University of Tanzania, where he has been a faculty member since 2006. Within his 15 years of service at the University, he has served several administrative positions as the Regional Director, Head of Economic Law Department and the current position as the Faculty Associate Dean. He holds a PhD degree from the Open University of Tanzania specializing in Mobile Money Regulations, Master of Laws degree specializing in Cybercrimes and computer Forensic Evidence, Bachelor of Laws (LLB) degree from the Open University of Tanzania, and Bachelor of Education in Science majoring in physics from University of Dar es Salaam. His research interests lie in the area of digital rights, cybercrimes, mobile money, artificial intelligence, land rights, and traditional knowledge. Abdallah has attended and presented papers at several local and international trainings, seminars, and workshops.

Dr. Udochu Eke is a senior lecturer in the School of General Studies, Michael Okpara University of Agriculture Umudike, Nigeria. He was among the 17 Shell Petroleum Development Company of Nigeria (SPDC) research interns in 2011/ 2012 internship research program. He is a Jerusalem pilgrim (JP) and has some international and local publications to his credit.

Dr. Leonard Emma holds a PhD in Social Work (University of Pretoria), MA (Dev. Studies) (ISS, The Netherlands), MBA (MANCOSA, SA), Post-graduate Diploma in Project & Programme Management, Cranefield College of Project & Programme Management, SA, 2005, and BA (Social Work). She has over 15 years of experience in the social welfare sector having worked in both the public and private sectors. Research areas include employee assistance programs, social policy, social entrepreneurship, and community development.

Ms. Mbetu Gamuchirai is a registered lawyer in the High Court of Zimbabwe and social activist who prides herself in striving for social justice. She holds a Master of Laws from the University of Stellenbosch, a Bachelor of Laws, and a Bachelor of Social Science in Politics and International Studies from Rhodes University. Ms. Mbetu has a deep interest in public policy issues and has varied work experience in the Human Rights, Youth and Gender Rights Advocacy, and Legal and Finance Sectors. She has worked in both the public and private sectors for regional NGOs, financial service providers, and a financial regulator.

Prof. Ananias Janet holds a PhD in Social Work (North-West University Potchefstroom campus, SA), Master of Arts in Social Work (UNAM), and Certificate in Social Gerontology (Karlstadt University, Sweden). She served as the Head of Department of Social Work and Senior Lecturer, with a wealth of experience of over 10 years in social work practice and education. She has a number of publications in scholarly journals and has presented papers at national and international conferences. Her research areas include Social Gerontology, Intergenerational caregiving; mental health; gender-based violence; substance abuse; Child neglect/fosterage; Refugees, mixed method research.

Dr. Kaumba Kennedy Mabuku serves as a police officer within the Namibian Police Force, boasting an extensive array of roles throughout his tenure. He has fulfilled duties as a police instructor for both fundamental and advanced police training, as well as assuming positions as an operational and administrative officer, and even a Regional Training Officer. In 2019, he took part in the review of the Namibian Police Force Basic Curriculum and played a pivotal role in crafting training materials for Police Managerial Competencies Training. His involvemen text ends to being a facilitator at the SARPCCO School of Excellence, wherein he participated in the review of the school's modules in both 2022 and 2023. Furthermore, he is deeply engaged in academia, overseeing research papers for Master's and Honours students at Stadio Higher Education. Notably, he also dedicates time as a part-time tutor at the Institute of Open Learning in Namibia and moderator at the University of Science and Technology in Namibia. Driven by his passion for security and peace, he has ardently advocated for the establishment of the Institute for Security and Strategic Studies of Namibia, a registered entity with BIPA. In conjunction with his advocacy efforts, he has contributed to journals and has presented a paper titled "Dimensions of Food Security in Sub-Saharan Africa: A Blind Road map to Agenda 2063" at a post graduate research seminar under the theme "Namibia Rising" at the University of Namibia. Additionally, he has shared his insights through various articles published in Namibia's daily newspapers.Educationally, Dr. Mabuku holds a Doctor and Master of Policing Practices from Stadio Higher Education and Southern Business School and He also holds Master of Arts in Security and Strategic Studies with the University of Namibia.

Dr. Awarab Marvin is currently a Senior Lecturer in the School of Law at the Faculty of Commerce, Management & Law at the University of Namibia (UNAM). He holds an LLD from the University of South Africa (UNISA), a Masters of Law (LL.M.) degree in commercial law from the University of Cape Town (UCT), a Bachelors of Laws (LL.B.), and a Baccalaureus Juris (B.Juris) degree both from UNAM. His research interests lie in the areas of commercial law, law of contracts, labour law and employment-related matters, company law, and corporate governance. He previously served as member of the Magistrates' Commission. He currently serves on various committees of UNAM and also a member of Namibia Institute of Corporate Governance (NICG). Over the years, Awarab has authored books in various areas of the law.

Ms. Ndapandula Monika Shifotoka is a PhD candidate at Shanghai University in China, with research direction in Media Education. She holds a master's degree in journalism and communication with majors in International Communication from the Communication University of China (2018). Moreover, she holds a Bachelor of Arts (Hons) degree in Media Studies with majors in Public Relations and Professional and Intercultural Communication from the University of Namibia (2012). Ms. Shifotoka worked as a civil servant for over seven years in public information, having worked for the Ministry of Information and Communication Technology in the Namibian Government. She has experience in social media management, coordinating public information, and event management.

Her research interests are Media Literacy Education, Digital literacy, and New Media Studies, and she is passionate about access to information. In January 2021, she joined the World Trade Organization (WTO) as a Young Professional, where she deals with information and external relations.

Ms. Frieda Omagano Shifotoka is a Doctoral of Law (LLD) candidate at the University of Pretoria, with her research focus being on Intellectual Properties (Copyrights, Trademarks, and Patents). She is currently an intern at the World Intellectual Property Organization (Switzerland). She is a current member of the United Nations Association for Southern Africa and Member of the International Intellectual Property Law Association. She has experience in academia, private sector, and public sector. She was part of the 2019 Editorial Board of the Student Law Review at the University of Pretoria. She holds an LLM (2014) degree in International Trade Law from the Stellenbosch University, South Africa. She further holds an LLB (Honors) (2013) degree from the University of Namibia and Baccalaureus (Law) degree (2011) from the same university. She has authored various articles published in books and in a regional journal. Her recent publication is entitled "The Protection of Geographical Indications: The Example of Namibian Products, in the African Journal on Intellectual Property Vol 3 No 2, 2019." Frieda Omagano Shifotoka, research interest: international trade law, intellectual property, international development, gender rights, human rights.

Mr. Malematja Stanley is an admitted attorney of the High Court of South Africa with a right of appearance in the High Court and is practicing as attorney at the Centre for Child Law, based at the University of Pretoria's Faculty of Law. He holds an LLB degree from the University of Johannesburg, an LLM degree (with a distinction for the mini dissertation) from the University of Pretoria, and a postgraduate diploma in Human Rights Law Advocacy and Litigation from the University of Witwatersrand's Nelson Mandela Institute. In 2020, Stanley was nominated as one of 200 young most influential South Africans by the Mail and Guardian. He is a steering committee member of the Southern African Human Rights Defenders Network. He has a strong passion for human rights and has expertise in Protest Law and Child Law. In 2015, Stanley was honored with two floating trophies: Centre for Child Law and Danie and Chrissie Dorfling after he was declared the overall winner of the Child Law National Mootcourt Competition.

Dr. Helao Tuhafeni holds Basic Police Training Certificate (Luiperd Valley Police College), Cert: Supervision & Man. (IPI Police College), NCPA, NHCPA, NDPA (PoN), B.Admin (UNAM), MPA (UWC), and DPA (UNISA). Former Senior lecturer in Department of Social Sciences, NUST; Former Associate Dean for Teaching and Learning in the Faculty of Human Sciences, NUST. He is a former secondary school teacher. Research areas include policing, administration, governance, ethics, safety and security, management, and global governance and politics. He is a former Police Officer, in the Namibian Police Force, an served as Station Commander and Police Policy Analyst. Served on Namibian Police Force Security Committee on VIPP Transformation. He served as a member of Namibia National UNESCO Programme Committee on Social Sciences, He served as Namibia National Mentor for Advanced International Training Programme on Inclusive political Leadership under Swedish International Centre for Local Democracy (ICLD). Former Information Officer at DoE (now, ECN) who introduced and implemented the first Voters Education Programme in Namibia. Helao authored a textbook on Role of Regional Councillors in Namibia.

Prof. Chikadzi Victor holds Doctorate in Social Work (University of the Witwatersrand), Master of Arts Degree in Social Development (University of the Witwatersrand), Bachelor of Social Work Arts (University of Fort Hare), Certificate in Life Coaching, trainer of trainers certification, and an Assessor certification. research areas include social protection, child protection, Indigenous Knowledge systems, social policy, social development, social entrepreneurship, qualitative research, sustainable livelihoods, marital therapy, community development, change management, and coaching.

www.ingramcontent.com/pod-product-compliance
Ingram Content Group UK Ltd.
Pitfield, Milton Keynes, MK11 3LW, UK
UKHW041837031026
15587UKWH00002B/833

9 781666 924831